FITNESS WITHOUT LIMITS

TRAINING TO BREAK THROUGH BARRIERS AND LIVE FEARLESSLY

FITNESS WITHOUT LIMITS

TRAINING TO BREAK THROUGH BARRIERS AND LIVE FEARLESSLY

BEN MUDGE

TEXT BY CAMILLE DEPUTTER

SPHERE

SPHERE

First published in Great Britain in 2024 by Sphere

1 3 5 7 9 10 8 6 4 2

A CIP catalogue record for this book
is available from the British Library.

ISBN 978-1-4087-3361-5

Designed by D. R. ink

Picture credits: All photos courtesy of Chris McCann except Adobe Stock Images on pages 30, 34–35, 69, 71, and 72. All illustrations courtesy of Emil Dacanay

Printed in China

The Mifflin-St Jeor Equation on p 63 is taken from Mifflin MD, St Jeor ST, Hill LA, Scott BJ, Daugherty SA, Koh YO., 'A new predictive equation for resting energy expenditure in healthy individuals', *The American Journal of Clinical Nutrition*, 1990;51(2):241-7. doi: 10.1093/ajcn/51.2.241.

Papers used by Sphere are from well-managed forests and other responsible sources.

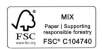

Sphere
An imprint of
Little, Brown Book Group
Carmelite House
50 Victoria Embankment
London EC4Y 0DZ

An Hachette UK Company

www.hachette.co.uk
www.littlebrown.co.uk

To my mum and dad,
thank you for everything you've done for me.
I'm lucky to be your son, love you.

CONTENTS

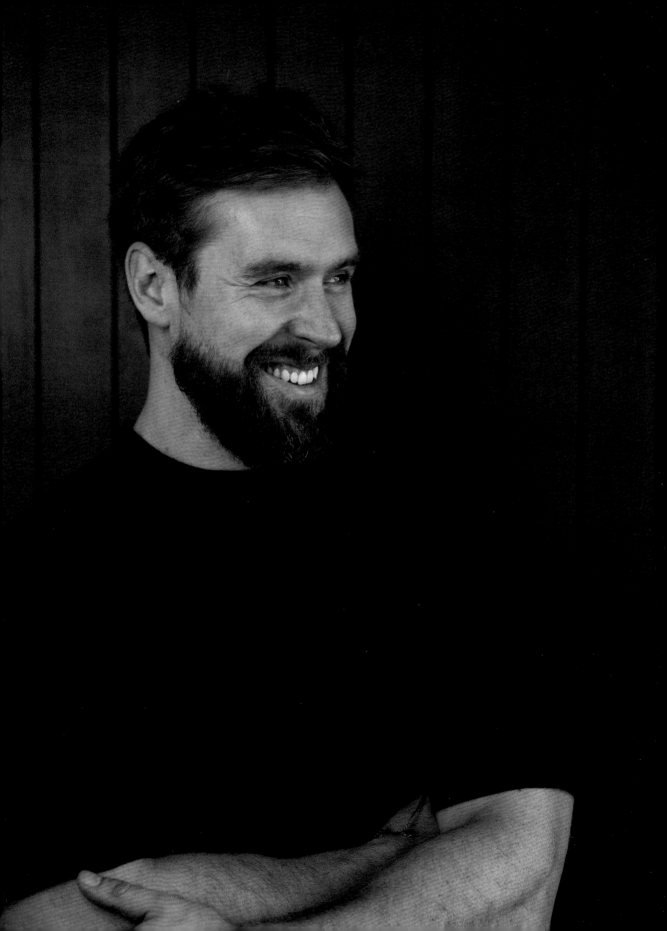

INTRODUCTION

O n a bright sunny morning in 1990, a woman stood outside the glass walls of the neonatal intensive-care unit in a Belfast hospital. A nurse, noticing the woman's gaze, pointed to a newborn baby who lay snugly in an incubator. Fresh scars dotted the infant's tiny body, the largest stretching from one side of its stomach to the other.

'Oh, that poor thing,' said the nurse. 'I feel so bad for that child's parents. That baby has cystic fibrosis. Life is over for those parents. They'll have oxygen tanks in every room. They won't be able to travel or put him into normal schools. He's basically a dead weight to that family.'

The nurse walked away. But the woman, who had been staring at her son, remained. That woman was my mum. And the baby, of course, was me.

This story still pains me. No parent should ever have to hear such things about their child. To be fair, at the time, the nurse's gloomy outlook wasn't off base. Back then, the outlook for cystic fibrosis (or 'CF') wasn't great. Even today, with some significant medical advances, cystic fibrosis is a potentially life-threatening disease that affects the respiratory system, digestive system and reproductive system.

Fortunately for my parents, and for me, the nurse was wrong. Growing up, while I did have other challenges, my lung capacity was hardly an issue – there were no oxygen tanks, thank goodness. I went to the same schools as my two siblings. We did occasionally travel as a family. Not to mention the other surprises and joys life has brought me: who would have guessed that I would one day become an award-winning bodybuilder, a fitness model, and the subject of a television documentary? I've gone surfing in Costa Rica, I've paddle-boarded from the Bahamas to Florida to raise money for cystic

> ## *As a child, without even realising it, there was a part of me that said:* No way. No way am I going to let my CF hold me back.

fibrosis, and I've used my likeness to superhero Thor to inspire children with CF. Best of all, I have a job I love. As a health and fitness coach, I help people all over the world to get stronger, fitter, healthier and happier.

Maybe, in a weird way, that nurse did me a favour. While I'm sure it wasn't her intention, she was placing limitations on me right from the start, declaring the boundaries of my potential just days after I was born. She was the first, but not the last person to define my limits for me. Sometimes I wonder whether these imposed limits sparked a kind of rebellion within my subconscious. As a child, without even realising it, there was a part of me that said: *No way. No way am I going to let my CF hold me back. No way am I going to miss out on all that life has to offer.* Right from the get-go, I was fiercely determined to live not just a 'normal' life, but a full, meaningful life. And I've always refused to let so-called limitations stand in my way.

That said, I still have to pinch myself sometimes when I look at what I've been able to experience and accomplish so far. Especially considering the fact that, while I had a relatively normal childhood, I was far from a prodigy when it came to sports and fitness. I was shy, small and not particularly gifted when it came to sports. Truth is, I was a big nerd – well, a *little* big nerd – growing up. My imagination was my strongest muscle, and I was more interested in video games than sports. That's not to say I didn't try. For example, at seven years old I played Saturday-morning football with my friends. (It was a tough choice between that and watching *Pokémon*, but somehow the football won out . . . most of the time.) I probably played thirty or forty games, and I gave it my best effort every time. But I only ever scored once.

At eleven years old, in secondary school, I started to play rugby. I really wanted to make the team, so I practised every single evening in our home garden, kicking the ball as high as I could and attempting to catch it over and over again, even as my hands got increasingly raw and sore, late into the chilly autumn evenings. Despite my best efforts, the coach usually kept me on the sidelines as a substitute. (And that's saying something, because we

Left: With my mum after my meconium ileus surgery

Right: My favourite homemade superhero costume

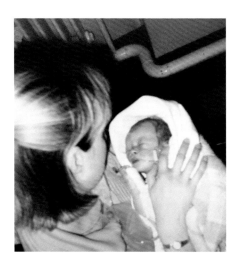
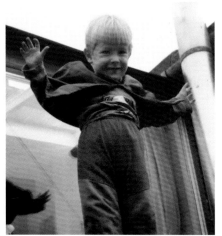

were not a good rugby school. Trust me on that.) I spent a lot of time on the sidelines with my dad, watching everyone else play, desperately hoping for an opportunity to prove that I was good enough to be on the team – but I rarely got the chance.

I was an active kid, always running around and playing with my older brother and friends. So it's hard to say why sports weren't my thing: did it have to do with my CF? Was there some kind of psychological barrier? I honestly don't know. Certainly, my parents never held me back or tried to discourage me from playing sports. I know a lot of parents who have children with CF, and the natural response is to bubble-wrap their children and protect them at all costs. Thankfully, mine didn't do that to me: they made sure I was safe, but aside from that, they let me be a kid. Further, my dad served as a remarkable role model by taking good care of his own health. He went through a simple workout every evening, consisting of push-ups, pull-ups and sit-ups. Naturally, I wanted to imitate him – he was my hero. By the time I was six years old, that little routine became so ingrained in me that I couldn't fall asleep without it.

While sports didn't interest me that much, by the time I turned sixteen, I was sick of being 'the small one'. I wanted to be bigger, more muscular, and – if I'm being completely honest – I wanted girls to like me. For Christmas, my parents got my brother and me a multigym (a big workout machine). I went through the manual and did every exercise that you could possibly do on the machine, and I kept at it. My efforts paid off; I started to gain muscle on my lean 59 kilo (130 lb; that's 9 stone 2 for my fellow Brits) frame.

It might not have been my explicit motivation, but getting stronger did help quiet the fearful little voice in my head: the voice that worries about getting sick, about being hooked up to oxygen tanks, about missing out on the long, full life I've always wanted. As I gained physical strength and size, my fear and worry seemed to shrink. This was my first taste of how empowering it can feel to take ownership over one's own health. Unfortunately, I would soon learn that the reverse is also true: it can be profoundly disempowering to lose control of your health and wellbeing. And there's nothing quite like the sheer terror of losing your most life-giving force – your ability to breathe.

At the age of twenty, while enrolled in a higher national diploma programme to pursue a career in the film industry, I noticed that something wasn't right. The first sign appeared on holiday. The moment my family arrived at our villa in Florida, I jumped into the pool for a swim. But as I dived underwater, I felt myself gasping for breath. My lungs couldn't seem to get enough air. I felt a twinge of worry, but brushed it off, chalking it up to the fact that I hadn't been particularly active recently.

When we arrived home, I raced up the stairs to my bedroom, which was on the top floor of our three-storey Victorian house. I always ran up as quickly as I could go, but this time I found myself panting heavily. Light-headedness washed over me the moment I got to the top. Once again, I tried to dismiss the reaction. But when the same breathlessness came over me the next day, I couldn't deny it any longer. I told my mum about my symptoms and before I knew it, I was sitting in the CF clinic being pumped full of intravenous antibiotics.

It turned out I'd acquired a chest infection. The doctors assessed my lung function at 66 per cent. (For context, lung function refers to what would be considered typical for someone of a similar size, sex, age and weight – without CF.) CF can affect lung function, and even cause respiratory failure. But that had never been my issue; rather, it was digestive issues that had plagued my childhood, which contributed to two hospitalisations with bowel obstructions. Growing up, my lung function typically came in around 100 per cent – in other words, normal.

This was new, and it was not a welcome surprise.

I made a pact with myself: **I will do absolutely everything I can to get healthy again, and stay that way.**

All I wanted to do was go home and hang out with my friends, but the doctor told me I couldn't leave the clinic until my lung function had improved to a tolerable degree. So instead of goofing off like a typical teenager, I sat woefully in a hospital bed, hooked up to scary-looking equipment and feeling like my entire life had changed in a flash.

One morning during my stay in the clinic, I woke up to a sound like I'd never heard before, coming from across the hall. I was certain it must be a machine: surely this wet, growling, grinding, hacking noise couldn't come from a human being. It sounded like Gollum coughing up a hairball. Every time I heard it, a chill went down my spine. Something about the noise was deeply unsettling.

I continued to hear it periodically, but I couldn't figure out what it was. Then, one afternoon, the door across the hall swung open. I leaned over to peek into this mysterious room. What I saw made my heart sink.

It was another room, just like mine. No machines. Just a nurse tending to a frail old man. The man was hunched over, his spine curved, his arms as thin as twigs, a wretched cough coming from deep within his lungs.

Until then, I didn't know a person could make such a sound.

Later that day, I walked past the man's room, where patient details were scrawled on a white board. I stole a glance and immediately wished I hadn't. The man was not a man but a boy – just a few years older than me. He, too, had CF. *Is this my future?* I thought. *Is this what lies in store for me?* I stumbled back to bed in tears.

These days, I think about that boy with deep sympathy and compassion. I truly wish he could have experienced a different outcome. But at the time, all I felt was fear and self-preservation. I really, really, *really* didn't want to end up like him.

At that moment, I made a pact with myself: *When I get out of here, I will do absolutely everything I can to get healthy again, and stay that way.*

After approximately two weeks, the antibiotics started to kick in and work their magic. My lung function was still poor (around 73 per cent or so) but good enough for the doctors to release me. It was finally time to go home. I had never been so happy to sleep in my own bed.

From then on, I kept my promise. In addition to going to the gym regularly, I worked diligently on my cardio. Before every workout I ran a mile on the treadmill. At the time, I hadn't quite cottoned on to the way other health practices like sleep, stress management and nutrition could play a role, but I knew for certain that prioritising cardiovascular health was a must. Slowly – very slowly – my lung function improved. Every three months I returned to the clinic to have it tested, and at each visit it was a little bit better.

Then, two years later, at twenty-two, just when I thought I was out of the woods, I came down with another chest infection. And this time it was worse.

Once again, I found myself sitting in a hospital chair, feeling like C-3PO, with my arms outstretched awkwardly, one stuffed with a long line IV, the other painful and taut with cellulitis after the first attempt at a long line didn't work.

Two weeks went by with no apparent improvement. Eventually, a visiting CF specialist knocked on my hospital-room door, an army of medical students in tow. They discussed my case at the foot of my bed without even acknowledging me, which made me feel a bit like a zoo animal. After ten minutes of this oddly one-sided interaction, I got fed up.

'What's going on?' I asked the doctor. 'Why am I still here?'

The specialist – the person who was supposed to be the foremost expert on my condition – answered bluntly, 'We don't know.'

'What does that mean?' I asked.

'The antibiotics don't seem to be working,' he replied plainly. 'We're monitoring your progress, but at this point, we're just shooting in the dark.'

'Does that mean I won't get any better?'

'You might not see much of an improvement,' he answered. And with that, he and the medical students filed out of the door.

And that's when I heard it. Another voice – my own, internal voice – coming from deep within.

Resolutely, the voice inside me said, *He's wrong.*

I trusted this voice. Something about what the doctor said just didn't add up. I knew I could feel better than this. After all, I'd improved my lung function and capacity before. Who's to say I couldn't do it again? With that decision made, I called the nurse and requested a stationary exercise bike for my room. I wasn't going to let my lack of freedom limit me.

The days dragged on, but I was determined to remain hopeful. And slowly, things did get better. Once my lung function hit 76 per cent – after fourteen days in the hospital – the doctors sent me home. I returned to life with a crystal-clear goal: I was going to restore my lung function to 100 per cent. I'd settle for nothing less.

Once again, I focused on building up my cardiovascular capacity. I started with cycling, and then graduated to short runs every morning. I began with 300 metres, then slowly, over the course of several weeks, graduated to 500 metres. Then to 700 metres, then to a kilometre. Bit by tiny bit, my lung function – and with it, my endurance and stamina – improved.

My progress was not a straight line. A few weeks after my hospital stay, while training with my friends in the gym, I suddenly felt submerged by fatigue. My brain was raring to go, but my body was telling me a different story. I sat down on a bench, disappointment curdling in my stomach.

Maybe I should just quit, I thought to myself. *This is embarrassing. This sucks. I've been doing this for ages, and I'm not making progress. It's going nowhere.*

I gazed at the rack of dumbbells that seemed to be taunting me. Before my hospitalisation, I could move them all so easily. But now, even the lighter weights felt like a struggle. My shoulders slumped.

Yet something shifted as I sat on the bench. Slowly, I got my breath back. My energy perked up just enough so I could get up and complete the rest of my gym session, making modifications as needed. It wasn't my best, strongest workout ever. But I got it done. I left the gym that day with a new promise to myself: to just keep showing up.

That remained my approach, day after day, week after week, month after month.

One year and ten months later, I returned to the clinic for yet another check. I did the lung-function test, my heart racing and my head pounding as I

As my clients worked towards their goals, I'd be right there with them – a fellow warrior in the quest towards health and fitness.

breathed into the little tube. I wanted nothing more than to see the number I'd been working towards for so long. I closed my eyes and repeated the same words to myself over and over: *Please let it be 100 per cent.*

And there it was.

I'd done it. My lung function was back to normal. It was the most rewarding feeling of my life. A wave of pride washed over me.

I may have reached my goal, but I knew the real work was far from over. It had become obvious to me that while other people might get to ignore their health – skip the gym, eat whatever they want, tell themselves they'll get around to taking care of themselves 'one day' – I didn't have that luxury. If I wanted to live a full life, my health had to be my number one priority.

Up until that point, I'd been dead set on a career in film, ideally as a director. But after my hospital stay, I knew that had to change. I needed a job that would allow me to take care of my health and wellbeing, and my few stints on film sets had shown me that directing was not compatible with that. Filming requires long, arduous days on your feet. It's a stressful job that can take a major toll on both your physical and mental health. I might have been disappointed, but it was as though a new path had revealed itself to me with perfect clarity. I knew I was going down a different road, and that was okay. Almost overnight I had a new goal, a new mission: I would become a personal trainer and help people get fit, healthy and strong. As I trainer, I could set my own hours and prioritise my own wellbeing, all while helping others live healthier, fuller lives. As my clients worked towards their goals, I'd be right there with them – a fellow warrior in the quest towards health and fitness.

From there, a whole new era of my life opened up. Over the next few years, I went down the fitness rabbit hole, getting my personal training certification and learning absolutely everything I could. At the same time, I remained steadfast with my own training, building up not only my cardiovascular fitness but also my muscle and strength.

While pursuing my new career, I worked at a local newsagent. Every day, during our slow hours, I'd flip through the fitness magazines, especially *Muscle & Fitness*, which boasted headlines like, '28 Days to Massive Arms' and 'Eight weeks to TREEmendous Legs'. I followed their programmes and, without realising exactly what I was doing, fell into bodybuilding-style training. By this stage I weighed 73 kilos (160 lbs) and had gained about 14 kilos (30 lbs) of muscle.

One afternoon at the gym, a fellow fitness professional started chatting with me. He told me about fitness modelling and physique competitions. 'Honestly,' he said, giving me the once-over, 'I think you have what it takes.'

Then he paused. 'Actually,' he added, thinking it over. 'The NIFMA (Northern Ireland Fitness Model Association) is having a competition in just two weeks. You should try it.'

Me, a fitness model? It seemed almost laughable. But there was a small seed of confidence growing within me. Could this once-skinny kid with CF become a competitive fitness model? Maybe it wasn't so crazy.

That very afternoon, I signed up. Somehow, I'd gone from being a kid in hospital with CF, to a bodybuilder and personal trainer. File that under things I didn't see coming.

Bodybuilding changed how I thought about my body – not just my physique, but my genetics. Growing up with CF, I'd always believed that my genetics were bad, they were working against me. But as I continued with bodybuilding, I came to realise that in some ways I'm genetically gifted. Many people don't realise that getting a 'bodybuilder body' – complete with round, bulging muscles that seem to pop out of a lean frame – isn't just a result of training. It's partly due to genetics. Some people have muscle insertions and muscle bellies, or muscle fibres, that are naturally more visible and will respond more easily to training. When I put in the work, my body responded with visible muscle development. For the first time in my life, my genetics were actually working *for* me. I like to joke that I may have been born with CF, but I was also gifted with some decent calf muscles.

Better still, CF wasn't part of the conversation. No one in the bodybuilding community knew or cared about my CF; they just wanted to talk about

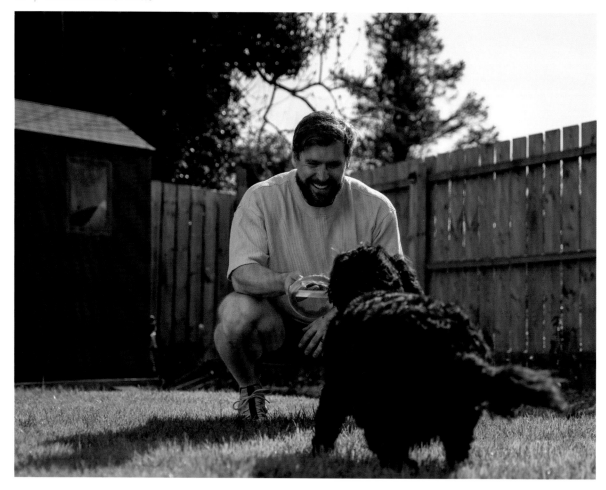

training methods, or nutrition protocols. And the further I could push CF away from me and the focus of my life, the better. For the first time, I didn't feel like I was a person with CF. I was just a person. A person with really good calves.

Over the next four years I continued with bodybuilding, taking some titles as I went. After winning the first men's physique competition in Northern Ireland, I was eligible to attend the British Finals at the United Kingdom Bodybuilding and Fitness Federation (UKBFF). This was a big deal because the winners of the British Finals would get their pro card and get a chance to compete at Mr. Olympia, the event that made Arnold Schwarzenegger famous. Unfortunately (or perhaps fortunately, depending on how you look at it), this event served as a wake-up call for me. I realised that I could never win at the international level with a natural, steroid-free body. Maybe I was naive, but it had never occurred to me that the vast majority of bodybuilders take steroids. This discovery soured my feelings about bodybuilding in general, but after some reflection (and an epiphany I'll tell you about later in the book), I decided I was ready to move on anyway. By this point, I was getting some attention based on how I looked. I'd been featured in some of the very magazines that I had read in the newsagent years before, and my story had gained interest on social media. It had been refreshing to build a name for myself without having to talk about CF, but it was all about appearance. And while I didn't want to be known for having CF, nor did I want to be appreciated solely for the size of my biceps. If I kept chasing the perfect bodybuilder's body, I realised, I would have a very empty life.

At twenty-five, I made the decision to retire from bodybuilding. At first, with this decision made, I floundered. My motivation to train lagged. In the bodybuilding community, I'd felt like I belonged. Now I had to ask myself: *Who am I? Where do I fit in? And what role does fitness play in my life?*

I wasn't sure how to answer those questions yet, but I knew there had to be more to fitness than just bodybuilding. So, I did what I'd done before: I learned everything I could. I expanded my educational horizons, completing additional certifications and attending multiple practical workshops. I discovered which kinds of training, nutrition and lifestyle practices deliver the best bang for their buck – not on the stage, but in real life, for the long haul. I explored different training modalities, and learned how to train for strength, functionality and injury prevention, rather than just muscle development. Going beyond exercise and nutrition, I researched things like sleep, recovery, stress management and good mental-health practices. And I invested in improving my practice as a coach, deepening my knowledge about behavioural change and how to develop lasting habits.

As my knowledge and understanding evolved, so too did my personal approach to movement, nutrition and overall health. I stopped training like a bodybuilder, and started to become more interested in how I was moving rather than what I looked like. Before, I'd followed programmes solely for the results, and whether or not I actually *liked* training was a non-issue. Now, I began leaning in to what I enjoyed. I felt like a kid again, having fun with my workouts.

I also started spending less time in the gym and more time doing things like walking my dog, Ollie, or going for a swim at the local leisure centre. As a bodybuilder, I used to train for at least two hours in the gym, five days a week. Now, I kept my sessions short and sharp. I spent time with friends and focused on getting a good night's sleep. My life became fuller, my days more pleasurable. Most importantly, I was able to maintain and improve my lung

One thing became crystal clear to me: there is no single 'right' way of doing things.

function and overall health. The base level of fitness I developed served as springboard for adventure and new opportunities: I was invited to take part in a physical challenge TV show called *Thru* (which was shot in Spain and featured contestants from all over the world), I took up flag American football and made the Ireland team, and I cycled 53 km on an assault bike for charity, just to name a few. I was even a contestant on an American TV show hosted by Dwayne 'The Rock' Johnson called *The Titan Games*; I was flown to Los Angeles to compete in the trials, testing my abilities alongside professional athletes, ex-military and other impressive individuals with exceptional physical fitness.

Through it all, one thing became crystal clear to me: there is no single 'right' way of doing things. Each person has their own journey. We each need to find what we enjoy, and what feels good to us. And when our preferences or abilities change, we need to be able to adjust. Rather than following a single programme, it's more about finding a path you can walk – with all its winding twists and turns – over the course of a lifetime.

Today, I can say that this approach has transformed my life for the better. Over the past decade, since my last hospital stay, I've remained healthy and strong. I'm grateful every day for the ability to breathe. And, without obsessing over muscle size, I'm a far cry from the skinny kid I once was.

Just as rewarding as caring for my own health is helping others do the same. Working as both an online and in-person coach over the past twelve years, I've helped hundreds of people from more than thirty countries achieve their own health and fitness goals. The vast majority of them aren't bodybuilders – far from it. They're people who want to keep up with their kids, people who want to feel better in a T-shirt. And for a lot of them, fitness has felt like it's been 'off-limits' for whatever reason.

Maybe you relate. Maybe you were the last kid picked for the sports team in secondary school; maybe you have injuries or illnesses that you're fighting; maybe you've tried every diet or training programme out there and it feels like nothing has worked; maybe it feels like you don't 'belong' in the gym or that fitness simply isn't for you.

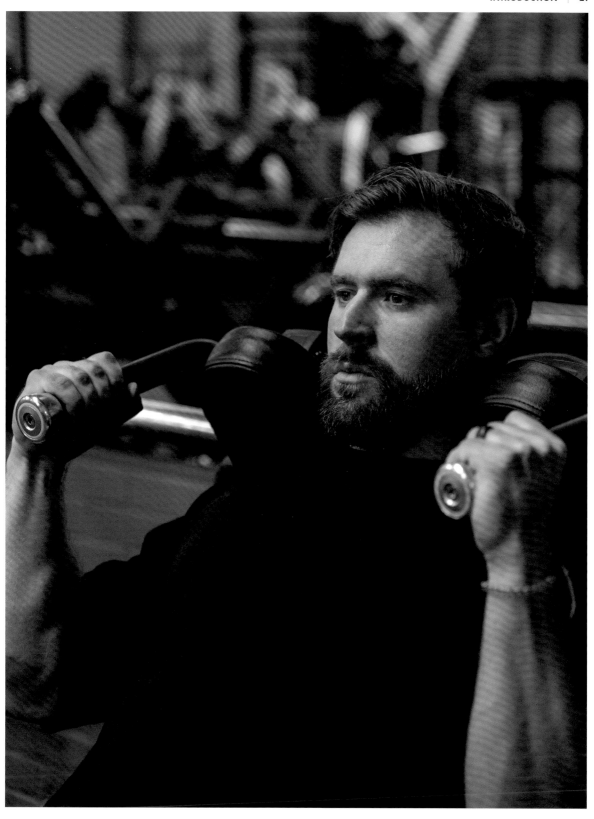

No matter your starting point, you can achieve any goal you set for yourself.

Whatever has got in your way or held you back, I get it. My story may be different, but I do know what it feels like to sit on the sidelines (literally and metaphorically) in life. And I can tell you this for certain: no matter your starting point, you can achieve any goal you set for yourself. (Well, within reason. You can't wave a magic wand and transform into the superhero of your choice. But I can almost guarantee that you can do more than you think you can.)

It is absolutely possible to feel better, to have more energy, to improve your strength and capability, to feel comfortable in your own skin. The best part is, you don't have to live like a bodybuilder to do it, eating only chicken and broccoli for every meal and spending over two hours in the gym every day. In fact, by adopting some relatively simple and sustainable practices, you can enjoy a far greater level of health, fitness and wellbeing than you've previously imagined for yourself. I've experienced it first hand, and so have my clients.

Take, for example, my client Lisandra. When Lisandra came to me, she was recovering from breast cancer. In her first session she was frail, wearing a hat to cover her hair loss, and she looked very tired. For our first session together, we went for a very slow five-minute walk. That was the most she could do back then. But I said to her, 'Don't get frustrated, this is just your starting point. You will only get stronger from here. I can't wait for us to talk about this moment in eight or twelve weeks' time. In six months, you won't believe how far you've come.' Lisandra nodded: she was committed. She knew what it was like to have her life threatened, to be on the verge of losing everything. Five months later, Lisandra was doing some of most rigorous cardio training sessions I could come up with and smashing every single one of them. Today, she's super healthy and I'm incredibly proud of her. More importantly, she's proud of herself.

Of course, this book isn't just for people who are battling a major health issue. So many people feel like health and fitness is somehow off-limits for them – like it's only for people who are *already* fit. The fact is, life can be tough. We all have our own challenges and obstacles; we all have our own dragons to slay. And that's why I've written this book: to help you in your quest, whatever your goal is. To help you conquer your challenges and come out on the other side.

In the first part of this book, you'll find a simple framework consisting of four core principles. This framework is built on the things that matter the most: practices that will offer you the easiest, most reliable gateway into a healthier and fitter life. You won't find absurd, unrealistic regimens here; instead, I will outline some core habits which you can adapt to your own life, no matter who you are or where you're starting from.

In Part Two, I'll dive into greater detail about exercise, and show you exactly how to integrate physical activity into your life in a sustainable way. I'll provide you with a scalable exercise programme you can easily modify based on your own needs, preferences, equipment and abilities. And I'll show you how you can complement your time in the gym with activities you actually enjoy, and simple habits that will fit seamlessly into the rest of your life.

Finally, in Part Three, I'll provide you with a programme-design tool, so you can continue to revise and evolve your workouts according to your tastes and abilities. Think of this as the 'pick and mix' of workouts.

By the end of this book, whatever limits you currently face will be left in the dust. You'll realise that you are far more capable than you ever imagined. You'll be better prepared than ever to take on new challenges and adventures, all while enjoying the benefits of glowing health, better energy, greater strength and the deep-down knowledge that whatever comes, you've got this.

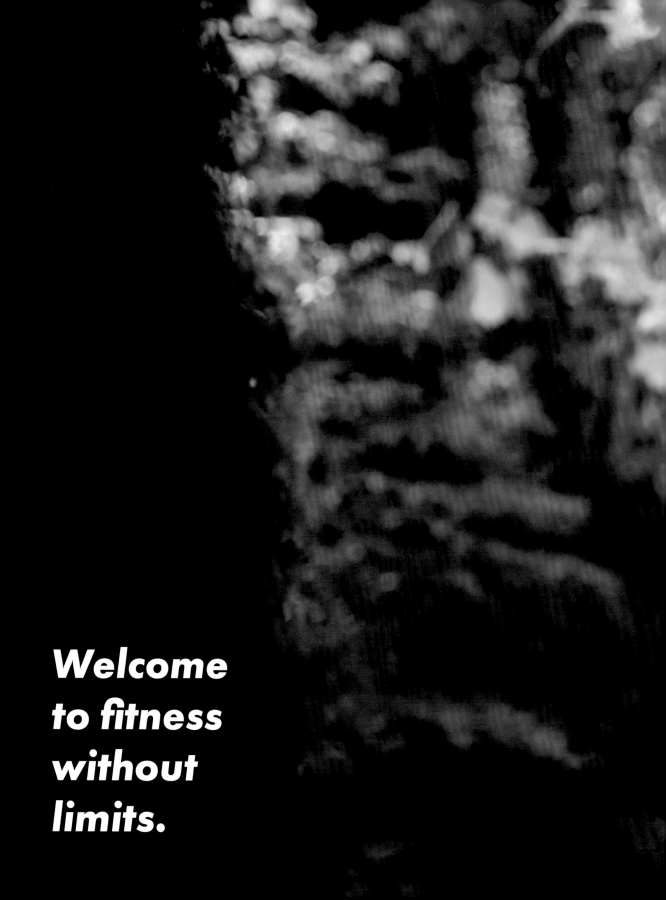

**Welcome
to fitness
without
limits.**

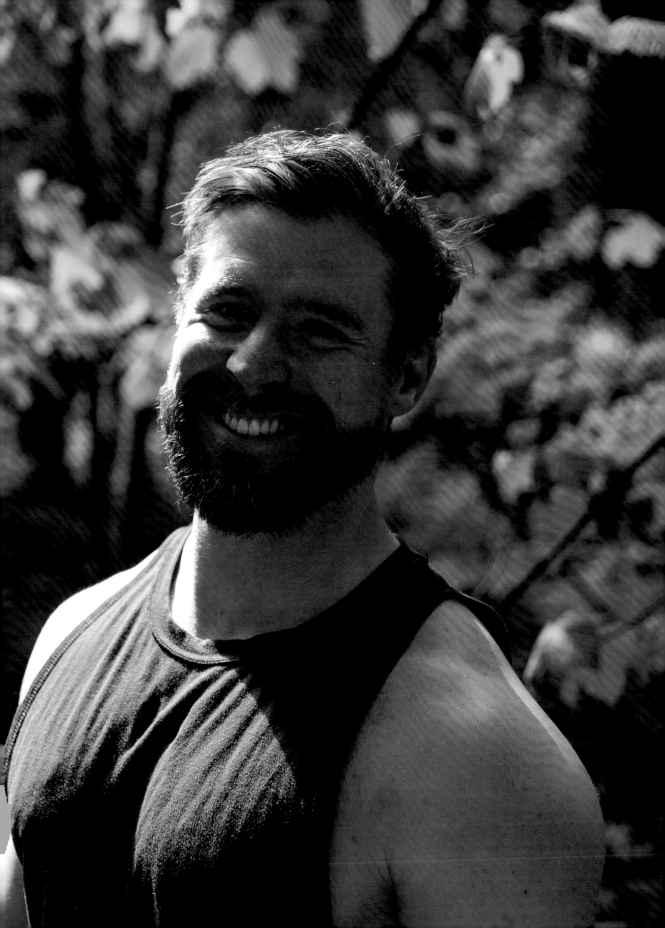

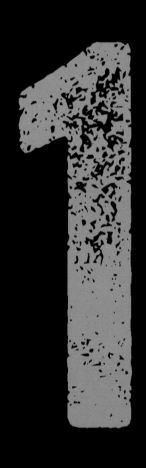

PART ONE

PRINCIPLES

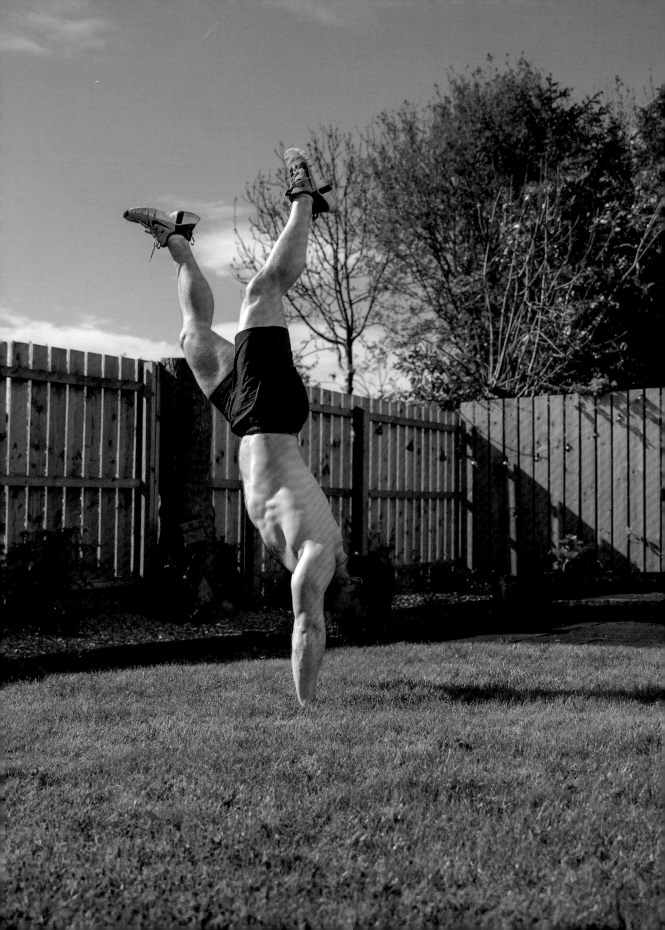

The amount of health and fitness information available to us these days is staggering. But when I take a step back and consider the things that have made a massive impact on my health and wellbeing (and that of my clients), it isn't that complicated. In fact, it all comes to down to four basic principles.

On the surface, these principles aren't particularly special. You might glance through the forthcoming pages and think, 'this is too easy', or 'that doesn't sound like enough'. And in fact, that's kind of the point.

Health and fitness practices *should* be simple. Think of it this way. When you choose to make an improvement in your life, you're essentially placing a bet on yourself: you're betting that you can do the thing you want to do. When you take on a convoluted, highly regimented fitness programme that you'll be unlikely to maintain (especially over the long run) you are betting *against* yourself. Why take that bet?

I want you to be 100 per cent confident that you will succeed. Commit to principles that you can do almost every day, over the long run – that's a winning bet.

As you'll see, I emphasise principles over a particular plan or detailed set of steps. If you follow these principles, you don't have to do them perfectly. You simply need to practise them in some shape or form, however small, over the course of your life.

You might conceptualise these principles as pillars. Imagine that your health and wellbeing is a beautiful building like the Parthenon. (I know the Parthenon has more than four pillars but it's always what I mentally picture because it has stood the test of time.) The pillars keep the building standing strong: without them, it would crumble. But with them, you'll remain steady: no matter what's going on in your life, no matter what challenges you're facing, these pillars will keep holding you up. And, while none of us are likely to last as long as the structures of ancient Greece, we can increase our chances of having a longer, better life.

Sure, you can always add to these principles. You can make the columns more intricate if you like, with more advanced nutrition or exercise protocols. But

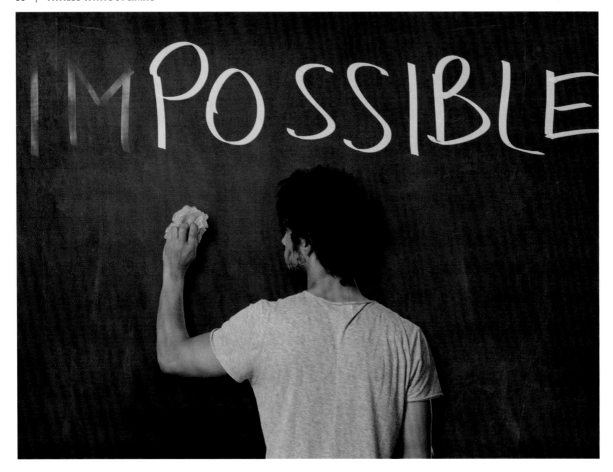

I promise, you'll get the biggest bang for your buck with these basics. And remember, they're your scaffolding. Without them, you won't have a building to decorate. Make sure you've got the core principles in place before adding more complexity.

For each of these principles, I've provided three practices for you to work on. Out of all the possible things you could do, these practices are the behaviours that will give you the best return on your investment of time and energy.

Before we dive in, here are a few foundational concepts to keep in mind. These are some general considerations that will help you implement – and reap rewards from! – everything you're about to learn.

You are a problem solver

Many people are reluctant to start exercising or improving their health in some way because all they see are obstacles or barriers to their success.

There's no doubt about it: You will encounter challenges and setbacks. Luckily, you're already a great problem solver. How do I know this? Because by picking up this book you've already identified something you want to improve in your life and you are taking steps to improve it.

The other reason I can so confidently say that you know how to solve problems is that you would not have got to whatever age you're currently at without navigating obstacles and challenges. That's good news because you can apply your existing problem-solving skills and methods to your health and fitness goals. Every time you run into an obstacle, consider how you might solve this issue in another context. If a friend or colleague were having this problem, how might you help them through it?

The secret to achieving fitness goals is not avoiding roadblocks. It's figuring out how to move around them.

Be firm with your goals, but flexible with your approach

When I set my sights on regaining my lung function, there were many days when I didn't feel like training, or I had poor energy. I knew that it was going to take months, maybe even years to achieve my end goal, and it would be impossible (and, honestly, undesirable) to train exactly the same way every single day for months on end. But I also knew that if I was willing to adapt my training – do a little more some days, a little less other days – I would get stronger over time, and eventually I would reach my goal.

There will be some weeks where you can't get to the gym. What will you do then? Perhaps you can do a bodyweight workout at home instead of your usual gym routine. Or if you can't do that, maybe you can go for a walk. Or if you can't do that, maybe you can turn on some music and dance around and get your heart rate up for the entirety of a single song. You read that right: dance around for roughly three minutes. That will be good enough some days. Trust me when I say that three minutes is better than nothing. Because the small things really do add up.

*All that is to say, don't depend on willpower.
Instead, focus on setting yourself up for success.*

Don't rely on willpower

Have you ever started your day feeling absolutely determined to do things 'right'? You begin by walking the dog and making the bed and ignoring the pastries that are passed around at work. As the day goes on though, something shifts. After some stressful meetings at work and a long commute home, your self-discipline starts to slip away. You wind up ordering a takeaway for dinner, downing a couple of big glasses of wine and snacking on biscuits or crisps in front of the TV. You go to bed wondering what the hell happened to all that willpower you started your day with. The reason is simple: willpower is a finite resource.

When it comes to self-improvement, people often try to summon their 'willpower' to make changes and stick to the goals they've set for themselves. But willpower (aka motivation) is finite, and it's easily depleted. To better understand how this works, imagine you're a character in a video game. Your game character has a limited set of health resources. (Like those little bars that show how much 'life' or 'health' you have left.) Every time your character gets hurt in some way, your health resources decrease, and if you don't replenish them, eventually you run out and it's game over. Willpower is a bit like those resources: you use it up. The more times you push yourself to do something you don't really want to do (like say, make a healthy breakfast rather than eat sugary cereals) you chip away at your willpower resources. That's why, by the end of the day, you'll feel less equipped to stick to the plan, and more inclined to throw your hands up and give in to whatever you feel like doing (or eating) in that moment.

All that is to say, don't depend on willpower. Instead, focus on setting yourself up for success. Pay attention to your environment, such as your home and workplace, and look for ways you can make healthy habits easier. At the same time, look for patterns that tend to derail you, and plan ahead to avoid potential roadblocks. In the coming pages, you'll see tips on how to do this. For example, when discussing sleep, I'll explain how to create an environment that is more conducive to a good night's rest. When exploring nutrition, I'll show you how to build in reminders to prevent yourself from forgetting your habits. And so on.

If you're not assessing, you're guessing

Quick: do you know exactly what you ate for breakfast, lunch and dinner three days ago? How about what you snacked on?

For most people, the answer would be no. And, even if you think you *do* remember, it's incredibly likely you're forgetting some detail. Maybe you remember the sandwich you had, but you forget having that second cup of tea or the random biscuits you munched on at your desk.

The human brain is a tricky thing. It's remarkable how much we can misremember things, or simply forget. Our guesses about our own lives (including things like our sleep, nutrition, movement habits and even our mental state) can be incredibly inaccurate.

This might not matter in your day-to-day life, but if you're trying to improve something, accurate data helps a lot. It's hard to know if you're making progress if you don't have a clear starting point, and a clear picture of your actions and behaviours. On the other hand, data can be a useful way of pinpointing which behaviours are working, which ones aren't, and exactly where you are (and aren't) making progress.

This doesn't mean you need an expensive smart watch, a pile of spreadsheets or a degree in health sciences. In fact, I think that getting obsessed with data can be detrimental if it takes your focus away from doing the key practices that matter most. As you read on, you'll see some options for collecting relevant data on yourself. I'll provide some slightly more advanced options for tracking as well as some basic self-assessments that anyone can do.

Start where the river is narrow

Imagine that you're going kayaking. First, you must assess the river to decide the best place to start paddling.

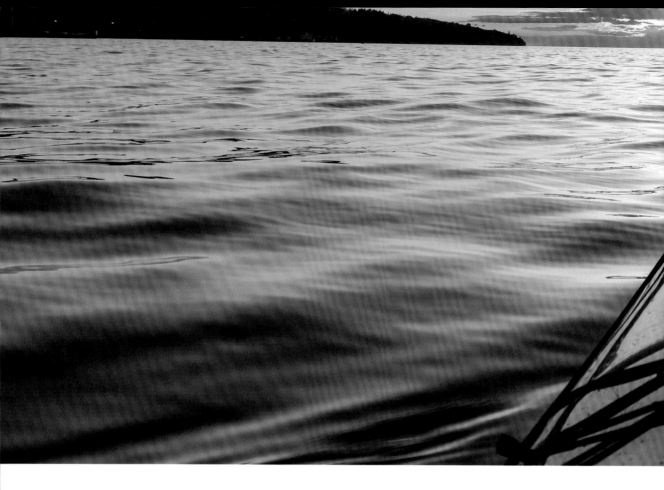

Where you currently stand, the river is narrow. It's tight and winding, and it won't be the easiest to navigate. You're a little nervous about making your way through all those curves. Further down the river, things open up. The river becomes much wider and calmer, so it's easier to navigate.

Where do you launch your boat? You might be tempted to choose the easier, wider part of the river. But my suggestion is to do the opposite: start where the river is narrow.

If you launch your boat where it's most challenging, you will figure out how to kayak through a tricky spot. You'll build the skills you need to kayak in a more difficult environment. When the river opens up, it'll be smooth sailing – great. But anytime you encounter a more challenging waterway, you'll know you can do it.

The same goes for training. If you have any sort of health and fitness goal, the best time to start is when things are stressful or busy. Because if you can figure out how to make progress when it's most challenging, you'll be far better equipped to keep going during whatever difficulties arise in the future. If you only learn how to do this stuff in ideal circumstances, you won't be able to keep at it when times get tough.

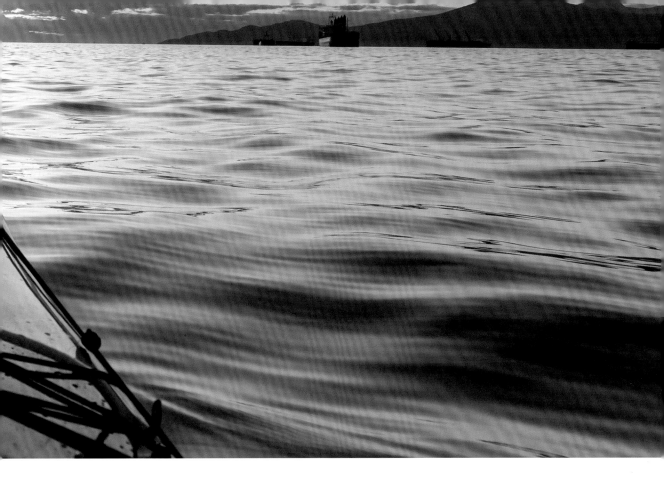

For a great example of this, consider my client Fatou. Fatou called me in the fall when she was busy working on a major project. 'I'm not ready now,' she told me. 'But I want to book you for the spring when I'll have more time.'

I told Fatou exactly what I'm telling you: that the perfect time to begin is now. I suggested we start working together and focus on small changes that would fit into her busy schedule. She agreed.

Fatou made lots of little improvements through our work. She ate more protein. She slightly increased her step count. Nothing that felt overwhelming or disruptive to her day. Over the course of sixteen weeks, Fatou noticed that her clothes fitted better, and she could comfortably wear jeans she'd previously chucked to the back of her wardrobe. Her overall fitness improved too. She noticed that she was no longer out of breath after going up a flight of stairs, and she was able to join her friends for the occasional morning power walk.

By the time spring rolled around, Fatou wasn't any less busy than she'd been in the autumn. As often happens with life, the 'perfect' time to train hadn't materialised. Yet Fatou had already made a ton of progress. Naturally, she was delighted that she hadn't waited to begin.

And you will be too.

Focus on principles and practices rather than goals

If I asked you what your plans are for this weekend, you might have an answer for me.

But what if I asked about your weekend plans for six weeks from now? Or twelve weeks? Or twenty weeks? Would you know exactly what you'll be doing then?

Likely not. It's hard for the human brain to imagine the future, especially in granular detail. And even if you happen to be great at dreaming up what you *want* to happen, you still can't know exactly what *will* happen. The further out you anticipate, the less likely you are to make an accurate guess of what's to come. That's one reason why people struggle with goals. The future is unknowable, and it's hard to have a deep attachment and commitment to something that feels distant, uncertain and maybe even unlikely.

That's not to say you can't or shouldn't have a goal. Go ahead and visualise the 'future you' that you want to achieve. But once you have that idea, shift your focus back to the present. Think about the steps that you can do *today* to make progress towards that goal.

I used this approach frequently in my own life. When I set my sights on getting my lung function back to 100 per cent, I asked myself: What do people with great lung function do? Then I focused on *doing those things*.

Similarly, when I wanted to become a fitness model, I asked myself: What do people who look like that do? How do they train, what do they eat? Again, I focused on *doing those things*.

I've applied the same approach to other hobbies, like Warhammer. For those who are less geeky than myself, this is a tabletop miniature war game that I've played since I was ten. When I started my Warhammer YouTube channel, I asked myself: what do successful people on YouTube do? You guessed it, I focused on *doing those things*.

In all of these instances, I knew what I wanted to achieve, but I didn't over-focus on the end goal. I paid most attention to what I could do each day.

Ideally, that focus on daily effort will be an enjoyable one – at least some of the time. If you obsess over some arrival fantasy – dreaming of how amazing it will be when you finally attain your dream body or life – but you're miserable during the whole process, I've got news for you: you will still be miserable when you achieve your goal. Conversely, if you enjoy the process – take pride in your efforts, celebrate small wins, give yourself a pat on the back for your hard work – your goal will be even sweeter when you achieve it.

There's an added bonus when you focus on the process, too. If you build practices into your daily life and make them part of your routine, they will eventually become easier. As you gain comfort and confidence, you'll stop feeling like your practices are something you *should* do and start feeling like they're something you *want* to do. They'll be more like a toolbox of supportive methods you rely on, rather than items on a to-do list. This is the real difference between people who work hard for a short-term goal (such as a crash diet) and the people who sustain a strong level of health and fitness throughout their lives – the people who truly live without limits.

Goals tend to be relatively short-lived efforts.

Principles and practices are for life.

PRINCIPLE #1: SLEEP

When I was twenty years old, my family went on a holiday to Florida. I'd planned on skipping the trip to work, but at the last minute my schedule cleared so I decided to tag along.

Unfortunately, since I hadn't planned on coming, the Airbnb my parents had rented didn't have enough bedrooms. On the first night, I slept on an airbed. Well, I *tried* to sleep, but the rubbery 'mattress' was old and full of holes. By morning it had fully deflated, and I found myself lying on the cold tiled floor.

The next night, I attempted to sleep on the sofa. I awkwardly tossed and turned, sweating and sticking to the leather upholstery.

The lack of sleep made me irritable and stressed, and the more stressed I became, the worse my sleep got. It was a vicious cycle. Still, I did my best to shrug it off. I thought I'd catch up on my sleep once we got home. But shortly after our holiday, my previous suspicions after swimming underwater were all but confirmed when I noticed it was harder to catch my breath. It turned out that I had come down with a chest infection, which wound up putting me in hospital. While I can't know exactly what happened, my guess is that I picked up a bug while travelling. Knowing what I know now about sleep and its impact on the body's ability to fight stressors and repair itself, I suspect that if I had been better rested, I could have fought off the virus I caught. Instead, it wound up putting me in the hospital for weeks.

Staying rested can help prevent illness and injury, but it's also so much more than that. Sleep is a cornerstone of good health. It's what allows you to move well, recover from your workouts, make good decisions that align with your goals, lose weight if you so desire, and generally feel good. Without sleep, you're pushing a boulder uphill. But give it the attention it deserves and you'll be amazed at what can happen. In other words, it is key to living the limitless life.

Take my client Brandon. Brandon was stressed out. He had a busy and demanding job, cared for his elderly father, and was heavily involved in community service. Despite everything on his plate, he was truly committed to losing weight and getting healthier. He arranged for a meal-prep service that ensured his nutrition was on point. He showed up for every workout religiously. He was doing so much 'right'. Yet despite some initial improvements, Brandon quickly hit a plateau. He just couldn't seem to make progress in the gym, or lose the extra weight around his mid-section.

At this point, I had a conversation with Brandon about his sleep. It turned out that he was up late most nights, tossing and turning, worrying about work, his father or things he'd seen on the news. As a result, he was only getting three to four hours of sleep per night. The impacts on his physical and mental health were starting to add up. I encouraged him to conduct a brain dump before he went to bed each night to help clear and prioritise his thoughts. (More about that technique in a bit.)

Brandon started to realise just how much his mental state was affecting his wellbeing. He'd been over-focusing on things that were well outside of his control, and it was preventing him from making progress. Eventually, he came to a decision. He shifted his focus to the things he could control, and put the worries out of his head. This single, deliberate choice allowed him to sleep. With some time and practice, he became a champion sleeper, getting in seven or eight hours each night.

After that, Brandon's results surprised even me – they were that impressive. He dropped 10 kilos (about 22 lbs or 1 stone 8 lbs) in roughly ten weeks. He returned to the gym with more strength and vigour, quickly adding weight to his usual lifts and busting out of his plateau. He'd been slogging away at his goals, and now, simply by getting more sleep, he achieved them almost effortlessly.

Brandon's story demonstrates why I get so excited about sleep – and hopefully, by the end of this section, you'll be just as excited as I am. In the coming pages, I'll make a case for why you should sleep more. And then I'll give you my top practices for getting better sleep.

Before we begin, I want to acknowledge that many people feel they don't get enough sleep due to circumstances beyond their control. Depending on your line of work, whether or not you have children (and how old they are), your age, health conditions you may have, and all kinds of other factors, you might struggle to get enough good, quality sleep. If that's the case, remember that perfection is not required. Aim for incremental progress. If you can improve your sleep just a little bit, or get a teeny bit more of it, I'd call that a win. One per cent is better than zero. In this section, I'll show you some ways you can make improvements with your sleep, without having to quit your job and join a monastery. Even if your sleep is limited, small improvements can do a world of good. Let's take a look.

Do less, sleep more

If I have my way, you won't see me in the gym before 11 a.m. This makes me a bit of an outlier among fitness professionals, who are generally known to be 'up and at 'em' types. Admittedly, I'm in the rare position of having lots of flexibility with my schedule. (And I don't have kids, which are pretty much guaranteed to interfere with your sleep, as any parent knows.) I take full advantage of this and sleep as much as possible. Lest you mistake me as lazy, let me assure you: this is a deliberate choice I make on behalf of my health.

Sleep might seem like a luxury, rather than something to practise and prioritise. If anything, most of us have been taught that getting fit requires less sleep, not more. Sleep is absolutely critical to good health, yet it's sorely neglected, even among 'fitness types'. You might see people boasting on Instagram about how they get up at 5 a.m. (or even earlier!) to exercise. Or you'll hear people bragging that they only need a handful of hours of sleep at night, quipping 'I'll sleep when I'm dead.'

(Please don't schedule sleep for when you're dead. When you're dead, you'll be dead. You're alive today, thank goodness, and that means you need sleep.)

Luckily, sleep is starting to get more attention and appreciation these days, as an abundance of research has shown that sleep is not only an important ingredient for feeling good, but also a legitimate, highly valuable component of health and longevity.

If you are struggling with your sleep, and you have to choose between improving your sleep or adding in exercise, I say: do less, sleep more. A good night's sleep makes *everything* else easier, which is why I prioritise it.

Why sleep matters

Imagine I could offer you a pill that would deliver the following results:

- ▶ Improved mood
- ▶ Improved cognitive function
- ▶ Stress relief and better mental health
- ▶ Regulated blood sugar
- ▶ Strengthened immune system
- ▶ Improved athletic performance
- ▶ Healthy weight (and fat loss, if desired)
- ▶ Healthy heart and vascular system
- ▶ Tissue repair and decreased risk of injuries
- ▶ Metabolic health
- ▶ Better relationships
- ▶ Increased energy
- ▶ . . . and more

Would you take it? Of course you would! Unless you were training for the Olympics – because you can be sure this magical pill would be a banned substance.

Sleep is basically a miracle drug. When you get plenty of sleep and have lots of energy, your potential truly becomes unlimited.

For an added plot twist, when you're not rested, you'll have less energy, making you less inclined to move and therefore burn fewer calories.

On the other hand, lack of sleep limits us in many ways. It's so much harder to push through any limitations (real or perceived) that you may have when you're not adequately rested.

Let's take a closer look at some of the reasons sleep is worth prioritising.

Sleep supports weight loss

We'll start with one reason that a lot of people care about: weight loss. If you're trying to lose body fat, or even maintain your weight, sleep is important.

A good night's sleep will help give you the mental clarity you need to make conscientious food choices, the energy you need to move well, and the recoverability to repair and build muscle after exercise.

On the other hand, lack of sleep can be detrimental to fat loss for a bunch of reasons. If you've ever had a poor night's sleep and then found yourself snacking endlessly all day or making less than ideal food choices, there's a reason for that.

Actually, a few reasons.

For one thing, without a good night's sleep, your cognitive function will be reduced – meaning you'll have less willpower to make smart food choices, and more inclined to make snap decisions. (As in, 'Aw, screw it, I'll have the burger and chips for lunch.')

Secondly, lack of sleep has an impact on your insulin levels, meaning your blood sugar will be elevated, leading you to crave carbohydrates and sweet snacks.

Thirdly, sleep makes a difference to your hunger hormones. Sleep decreases the hunger hormone, ghrelin (or as I prefer to think of it, *gremlin*, because ghrelin is like a little gremlin making your stomach growl). At the same time, sleep increases leptin, the hormone that helps you feel full. Without sleep, the reverse equation happens: more 'gremlin' + less leptin = more munchies.

For an added plot twist, when you're not rested, you'll have less energy, making you less inclined to move and therefore burn fewer calories.

You can start to see why, when it comes to building or maintaining a healthy body composition, sleep is your friend.

Sleep supports muscle repair and recovery

Have you ever lifted weights and noticed that your muscles immediately appear bigger? This is not your muscles magically growing before your very eyes. In fact, it's what's known as the 'lactic pump' – or in more scientific terms, transient hypertrophy. When you work your muscles hard, lactic acid builds up and draws water to them, temporarily causing them to appear bigger. (By the way, this is an insider tip used by fitness models: one of their many tricks is to pump up their muscles a bit by working them out just before having their photos taken.)

In fact, your muscles do not grow in the gym. When you exercise, you're actually breaking down your muscle fibres. When you rest and recover – i.e. when you sleep – they repair themselves and in doing so, grow a bit bigger. If you want bigger, stronger muscles, sleep is imperative.

Sleep also supports other types of recovery for different systems within your body. For example, it allows your nervous system to reset for the next day, and it boosts the body's immune system by helping to reduce stress and supporting the cells that fight off infections and viruses.

Sleep is necessary for good mental health and cognitive function

Imagine you're enjoying a nice cup of coffee in the morning when your partner or child wanders past you. Instead of saying 'good morning' or giving you a hug, they shuffle past you with a big scowl on their face, their grumpy vibes clouding up the room.

What do you say to them? Probably something like, 'Someone woke up on the wrong side of the bed this morning.'

We know that lack of sleep affects our mood and mindset. It's hard to feel chipper in the morning if you've barely slept – let alone if you're chronically underslept. Without sleep, even small issues or little decisions (like what to make for dinner) can feel like impossible hurdles. And if you have a mental health disorder, lack of sleep can make your symptoms worse. Conversely, when you're well-rested, you're better prepared to tackle whatever stressors you face, and make good decisions that support your goals.

Let's be honest: self-improvement is already an uphill climb. If you're not sleeping, you're putting lead boots on, making the climb so much harder than it needs to be.

Think about it like this. Stress is always going to happen – it's part of life. But when your recovery (in particular, your sleep) is greater than your stress, you'll be equipped to handle whatever comes your way, and still feel relatively good. This is what I mean when I say sleep is key to the limitless life. Sure, whatever limitations you're currently facing will still be there. But your capacity to handle them, challenge them and work around them will radically increase. They won't feel so big or unwieldy any more. That's why sleeping is like giving yourself a superpower.

Your ability to handle stress depends on your level of recovery. The higher the stress level, the more recovery you need. If you're facing stressors that are outside your control, increasing your level of recovery by sleeping more is an excellent strategy.

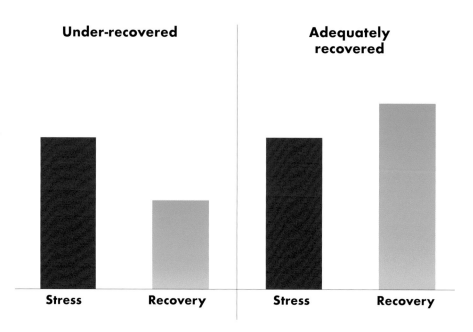

Under-recovered

Adequately recovered

Stress   **Recovery**   **Stress**   **Recovery**

How much sleep is necessary?

Research suggests that most adults need seven to nine hours of sleep a night. However, this kind of number can feel stressful to some. Depending on your situation – such as your job, whether you have small children etc. – getting eight hours of sleep a night might be impossible. Furthermore, you might find those numbers don't quite apply for you. Some people really do feel well rested with six hours of sleep a night.

What really matters is not what studies show, but how you *feel*. Improving sleep isn't about hitting some external target, but arriving at a place where you consistently feel rested and energetic.

To gain a better understanding of your sleep patterns, I encourage you to track your sleep. There are plenty of apps and tools on the market that can assess sleep quality and quantity. Or, if you prefer a simpler method, you can assess whether you're getting enough sleep by asking yourself a few simple questions:

- Do I generally feel well rested?
- Do I have adequate energy to do the things I want/need to do throughout my day?
- Do I bounce back and recover from my workouts within a day or two?
- Do I feel like I'm getting enough sleep for me?

I recommend asking yourself these questions on a regular basis (ideally daily) for at least a couple of weeks as they will help you get a better read on the state of your sleep. Write down your answers in a journal or notebook so you can review your progress.

If you consistently answer 'yes' to these questions, you must be doing something right! But if you answer 'no' to some or all of them, then it's probably a good idea to work on improving your sleep in some way. Remember: that doesn't mean it has to be perfect. Just aim for a little better.

With that in mind, here are some practices to help you improve your sleep.

Sleep practices

My three key practices to help you get a better night's sleep are:

- Establish (and follow) a sleep routine
- Attend to your physical environment
- Attend to your mental environment

Let's look at each practice, one-by-one.

Practice: Establish (and follow) a sleep routine

For many people, sleep is erratic. They might go to bed early on Sunday night and wake up early Monday morning; stay up late Wednesday night to catch up on work and still have to get up early for that meeting; and then stay up even later on Friday night and lie in on Saturday. You get the idea: their sleep is all over the show.

This system (or lack thereof) does us no favours. The simple fact is, people tend to sleep better, and generally feel better, when they go to bed at roughly the same time each day, and get up at the same time each day.

Sure, there might be some exceptions. (No one is stopping you from a night out at the weekend.) But generally speaking, you want to aim for some level of consistency. Here's how to make it happen.

Go to bed at roughly the same time every day

In some ways, sleep is like a debt collector. You might be able to ignore it for a little while, but it will catch up to you eventually – and demand interest. However, unlike a debt collector, you can't just pay off the debt and move on. If you drag yourself through the week (or weeks on end) with inadequate sleep and hope to catch up on the weekend, you'll find that you still feel depleted. Worse still, you may have trouble falling asleep at night, and difficulty getting up in the morning.

Consider when you typically have to get up in the morning. Then, plan to go to bed with enough time to feel rested by morning. For example, if you feel best with eight hours of sleep, and you have to get up at 7 a.m., plan to go to bed about nine hours in advance, at 10 p.m. That gives you some time to fall asleep and to account for potential sleep disruptions. 10 p.m. becomes your standard bedtime, and 7 a.m. becomes your standard wake-up time.

The 3-2-1 method

While you can't control sleep, you can do some things to help facilitate it. I call this the 3-2-1 method. Make this method part of your routine and you'll find it becomes easier to fall and stay asleep. Here's how it works.

Three hours before bed: Stop eating.

Ever notice that it's hard to sleep after a big meal? Aside from maybe feeling uncomfortable or bloated, when your body is digesting food your core temperature rises, which causes wakefulness. A key component of quality sleep is a drop in body temperature, so this makes your good night's sleep more difficult to achieve.

To avoid this, aim to stop eating three hours prior to bedtime. Using the example above, if you plan to go to bed at 10 p.m., aim to have finished dinner by 7 p.m.

Again, I'll remind you that this doesn't have to be perfect. If you're hungry and want a small snack at 8 p.m., have it. Simply aim to get close to the three-hour mark as often as you can.

Two hours before bed: Reduce fluid intake.

There's nothing worse than having to force yourself out of your cozy bed at 3 a.m. because you need to pee. Waking up in the middle of the night to pee is not only annoying – it interrupts your sleep pattern. The more often you have to get up, the worse your sleep will be.

This isn't always preventable: for example, if you're pregnant or perimenopausal you're likely going to have some unavoidable trips to the toilet, and that's okay. But for many people, simply drinking less before bed can make a difference.

Make sure you drink enough water through the day, and then taper off as you are about two hours out from sleep. Once again, make this habit work for you: if you're thirsty, go ahead and have a glass of water. But maybe skip the extra-large cup of tea as bedtime approaches.

1

One hour before bed: Step away from the screens.

To prepare for sleep, you'll want to reduce your exposure to blue light – the kind that emanates from our computers, phones, tablets and televisions. (More about light exposure in a moment.)

One hour before bed, turn off your screens. Try reading a book or listening to music as a 'wind down' instead.

Fair warning: this can be a challenging habit to break, especially if you're used to watching TV or scrolling through Instagram right until the moment you nod off. But it's worth it!

Practice: Attend to your physical environment

If you've ever tried to sleep somewhere really uncomfortable – say, on a deflated air mattress – you already know that your physical environment can play a role in your sleep. Yet many of us don't think to make our own bedrooms into restful spaces. They can easily become a catch-all: a place for storing baskets of laundry, watching TV, doing work or hiding miscellaneous messes when the in-laws come over. (Or is that last one just me?)

If you want to sleep better at night, attend to your physical environment – i.e. your bedroom. Aim to make it cool, dark and peaceful.

Keep it cool

To get deep, restful sleep, your body temperature needs to drop. That means you're better off sleeping in a cool room than a warm one. A cooler room will allow your body to come to an optimal temperature for both falling and staying asleep. Before bed (perhaps as part of your 'one hour before bed' ritual), turn the thermostat down a couple of notches. Set yourself an alarm if you need a reminder. If that isn't an option, invest in a fan or open a window.

Keep it dark

If you've ever been camping deep in the woods, away from all sources of light pollution, you know how incredibly dark it can get at night. This is how our caveman ancestors slept, and our sleep needs haven't changed. Darkness tells our bodies that it's time for bed. But small sources of light – particularly

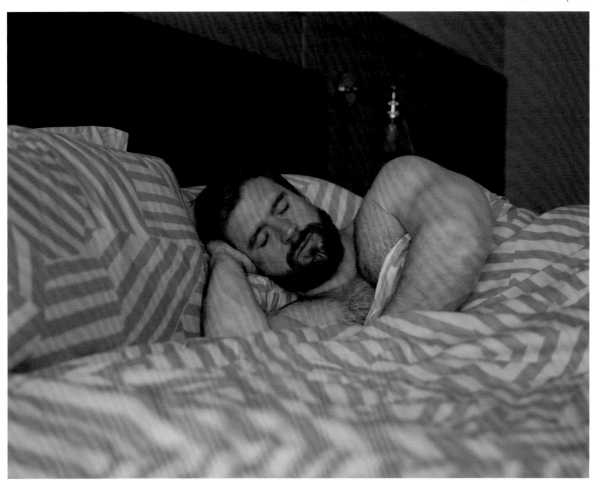

artificial light, like the kind coming from computers and other electronic devices – disturb our slumber and can make us more prone to waking up or sleeping lightly, which means we don't get the deep sleep we need. Even small sources of light can cause a bigger disruption than you might realise. To help with this, make sure electronics that have a light source are plugged into a different room or aren't visible. Additionally, try wearing an eye mask at bedtime, or consider investing in blackout blinds.

Keep it peaceful

It's pretty intuitive that a peaceful, well-organised room is much more conducive to sleep than a cluttered mess. A calm, well-kept room helps cue your brain that this is a place for rest. I don't want to sound like a nagging parent (yes, Mum and Dad, you were right!) but make your bed in the mornings and set aside some time each day to tidy away your stuff. Make sure your room feels pleasant and welcoming before bedtime.

Practice: **Attend to your mental environment**

Have you ever hurried around all day long, putting out one fire after another, and then collapsed into bed exhausted and anxious to sleep – only for your mind to keep racing? Try as you might, you can't seem to calm it down and fall asleep?

This is totally normal. Our minds need to unwind and settle in order for us to have a pleasant, peaceful sleep.

You can think of this as your mental environment. Just as a calm and well-organised physical environment can help facilitate sleep, so too can a calm and well-organised mental environment. Here are a few tips to help you prepare your mental environment for a good night's sleep.

Warm up (or cool down) for sleep

When you hit the gym, do you walk straight into the squat rack, load up the bar and start squatting? I hope not. Most people will do at least a brief warm-up before moving into a heavy workout. We should apply this concept to sleep as well. Just as you would warm up your body before movement, you need to 'warm up' – or perhaps more accurately 'cool down' – before sleep.

Consider designing your own cool-down routine. Some ideas could include dimming the lights, putting on some relaxing music, setting out your clothes or anything you'll need first thing in the morning, drinking some caffeine-free tea (not too much if you're less than two hours away from bedtime), reading some light fiction or writing down some things you're grateful for. Take some time to experiment and find the right blend of activities that work best for you.

Empty the washing machine

Many of my clients say the biggest problem they face when trying to sleep is that all their thoughts come at them at once. The moment they try to rest, their brain starts reeling with a whole bunch of thoughts, feelings, worries and concerns. Here's a trick to counteract this.

Think of your brain as a washing machine. If you've only got one red sock in the washing machine, it's pretty easy to see that sock going round and round. But if the washing machine is packed with clothes, it's hard to observe what's in it. You just see a big jumble of stuff.

This is what happens to our brains when they're packed with competing thoughts. Trying to pinpoint a single thought, consider it and then put it aside becomes tricky (if not impossible) when there's too much in there.

Unpacking your thoughts – pulling out the clothes and emptying the washing machine – can help. To do this, try the following exercise.

In a notebook or on a piece of paper, write down all the competing thoughts in your brain. Put it all down: no matter how silly or random any given thought may be.

Now, on another page, organise your thoughts. I like to use a grid known as the Eisenhower Matrix.

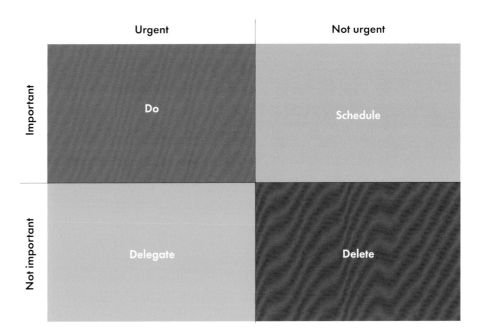

Using this matrix, you'll create a simple grid. Categorise each thought according to whether it's important or not important, urgent or not urgent. (I highly recommend writing this down in a notebook or journal; writing it out works much more effectively than trying to make sense of it all in your head.)

Once you've categorised your thoughts, you can see which ones require more attention. Don't worry about the stuff that isn't urgent or important;

put those issues aside for now. For anything that is urgent, important or both, write out a brief action plan for how you will tackle the issue.

I find this can be a useful end-of-day exercise. It minimises the thoughts competing for space in your brain and gives you a course of action for the most pressing priorities, which 'Tomorrow You' can take care of. It gives your brain a clear message: now it's time for sleep.

Summary

There are so many aspects of self-improvement that take work: going to the gym, shopping for and cooking healthy food, making deliberate choices about how you spend your time and energy. This stuff can be great – and truly, throughout this book I'm hoping you'll fall in love with the process – but it does require effort.

Sleep, on the other hand, means you get to lie down, close your eyes and relax. Aside from a little preparation and planning, it requires you to do, well, nothing.

Of course, as you've learned, while you sleep your body is busy with some very important processes of its own. Sleep is like a magic pill that will deliver a host of benefits, including helping you lose weight, get stronger, and feel more capable, energetic and – dare I say it – happier, as you go about your day-to-day life.

 RECAP

Your key sleep practices are:

● **Establish (and maintain) a sleep routine**
● **Attend to your physical environment**
● **Attend to your mental environment**

PRINCIPLE #2: NUTRITION

When I was twenty-one and getting into bodybuilding, I hired a coach to help me to get ready for my first photo shoot. The first thing he had me do was track all my food and beverages for a week. When I handed over my tracking sheet, he took one look at it and said, 'You have no idea how to eat, do you?'

'No,' I responded. He was right – I didn't have a clue. My meals were pretty random. For breakfast I might have a big bowl of sugary cereal, and for dinner a big pile of microwaveable chicken wings. My diet was not exactly refined.

Like I said, I was just twenty-one at the time. I had both limited cooking skills and limited funds. None of this seemed to matter to my coach, though, who presented me with a detailed meal plan that included steak with nuts for breakfast (you read that right) and 'fresh, line-caught salmon' for lunch.

I looked at that meal plan and thought, *What on earth am I supposed to do with this?* I may have been uneducated when it came to nutrition, but I knew that plan was not realistic. I attempted to follow it as best I could, but not surprisingly, I gave up after a week.

That's what usually happens with meal plans. People try them for a while, then quit. And with good reason: even the 'best' advice or carefully structured meal plan is useless if it doesn't work for you and your unique situation.

Humans are highly individual, and life is dynamic and ever-changing. Even if a meal plan is more down-to-earth than the one I received, it's unlikely to work for an extended period of time.

Getting a meal plan is like getting the answers to a test you didn't study for. You might pass the test, but you didn't learn anything – and you won't know what to do with the information once you've left the exam room. On the other hand, if you're able to integrate some simple yet essential practices into your life, you can maintain them no matter what comes your way.

And that's really the goal – to eat well, over the long term. When you give your body the energy it needs by eating mostly nutrient-dense foods (especially protein and fibre, as I'll discuss shortly), you'll be amazed at how good you can feel. As you likely already know, nutritious food supports good health over the long term. Eating a balanced diet of mostly minimally processed whole foods can minimise risk of illnesses and disease including cancer, heart disease and diabetes. It can boost immunity, support healthy bones, muscles, teeth and organs, and contribute to a longer life. Chances are, these facts won't surprise you. But if you're not used to eating nutritious foods in appropriate amounts, you might not realise how good it can make you feel. Eat according to the principles I'm about to share with you and you'll experience better energy, more strength and better recovery, improved sleep, better mood and mental health, and better digestion. Plus, if you have body composition goals such as fat loss or muscle gain, and/or performance goals, nutrition will play a pivotal role. Your goals will become much more achievable.

Many people are used to thinking of nutrition as setting limits – diets, restriction and so on. But nutrition doesn't have to be a limitation. Quite the opposite. It can be incredible tool to help you feel your absolute best, smash your goals and improve both your longevity and quality of life. Who wouldn't want that?

In this section, I won't tell you what to eat or not eat. What I will provide are some core practices and tactics that will enable you to eat in a way that supports your goals *and* aligns with your lifestyle and personal preferences.

Memories over muscle

Before we get into the nuts and ~~steak~~ bolts of nutrition, there's an added concept I want you to keep in mind. I call it 'memories over muscle'.

Let me explain what I mean with a story. Back in my bodybuilding days, I was considered an outlier because I seemed to get away with eating more (and with more flexibility) than some of my peers. Bodybuilders tend to be quite strict with their nutrition. Many will undergo highly restrictive diets for as much as sixteen weeks ahead of a competition or photo shoot. This is usually followed by a rebound phase where they'll eat anything in sight, gorging on pizza, pasta, doughnuts and so on. I tried to avoid this cycle as much as possible . . . but I wasn't totally exempt from it.

Truth be told, my eating habits were still fairly rigid by normal standards. My most restrictive diet, in advance of a competition, lasted 'just' seven weeks. Compared to my peers, seven weeks was nothing – but it certainly felt like a long time to me.

About five weeks into the diet, I was hanging out at home with a few of my housemates. By this point, I was in an extreme calorie deficit, and my body was feeling the effects. I was cold all the time, had low energy and was preoccupied by thoughts of food. As we sat around the living room, my nose twitched. I caught a slight whiff of a delicious scent in the air.

'There's peanut butter in here,' I said.

My friends looked at me like I was crazy. 'What are you talking about?'

'Trust me,' I said, and proceeded to root around through the kitchen cupboards.

Just as I suspected, one of the cupboards held a sealed jar of peanut butter. One of my housemates must have bought it. I grabbed a spoon and, with my housemate's permission, gently skimmed a thin layer off the top and ate it, savouring every bit.

Did I mention that I don't even like peanut butter? I think this story shows how extreme dieting can get to you. The more you restrict food, the more food-obsessed you can become. (Whether or not it can give you a dog-like ability to smell peanut butter is another story.)

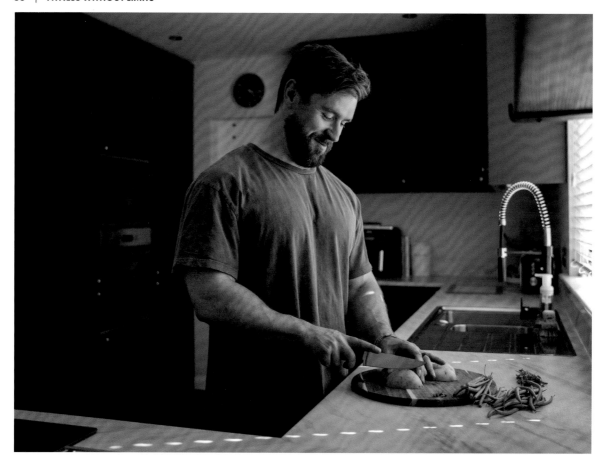

I knew the dieting would be temporary. What I didn't realise was how insidious it would become. The more time I spent in bodybuilding circles, the more anxious I became around food. And the worse I felt about my body.

At twenty-five I was featured on the cover of *Men's Fitness* – a magazine known for displaying bodies that most guys would consider aspirational. However, the photo was taken after I'd completed a bodybuilding competition and was already in a rebound phase. While the magazine publishers thought I looked cover-model fit, I saw myself as soft and squishy. Looking back at that moment it's sad to think that I felt embarrassed by the cover when the issue came out.

The epiphany came on my honeymoon. My amazing wife, Janice, and I lounged by the pool in Greece. I should have been relaxing but I couldn't stop worrying about how I looked. I felt self-conscious with my shirt off because my abs were not popping in the way they did when I was competition ready. These critical thoughts prevented me from being truly present and taking in the moment.

I excused myself from the pool and went back to the room to shower and change. That's when it happened. I stood in front of the mirror and looked myself in the eye. I felt a sudden shift, as though someone had slapped me on the back of the head. Out loud I said, 'What are you doing to yourself? Why are you taking away all the hard work you've put into getting strong, healthy, and fit? When you were fifteen, freezing your ass off in that garage gym you would have never believed that you would feel or look like this. You should be congratulating yourself for what you've achieved instead of critiquing every single thing about your physique.'

I decided then and there that I was done with trying to look better. Done with the negative self-talk. And done with bodybuilding.

To be fair, I was not alone. Body image issues are commonplace for bodybuilders and fitness models. People within this community are constantly evaluated based on how they look. Their bodies are scrutinised and closely compared. In bodybuilding and fitness model competitions, you are literally being judged on the exact size and shape of each of your muscles. Needless to say, this is an unhealthy way to live, and it can take over your whole life.

Of course, it's not just people on the stage who suffer from these kinds of concerns; many people do (maybe even most people). I was fortunate to have a moment of clarity that day. I want to live every second of my life with presence and appreciation, not spend it obsessing over my body or what I can or can't eat. And I want the same for you.

These days, I don't diet or follow meal plans, but I do maintain a couple of simple practices that help me feel energetic and strong, support good health markers, and maintain muscle mass . . . perhaps to the point of unbelievability. I recall visiting the CF clinic one day, where I caught a nurse eying me sceptically. Finally she admitted that she couldn't believe I could be this muscular without the use of steroids. I tried to educate her on the power of protein, but I still don't think she got it. To me, this speaks to how most people – even health professionals – misunderstand the power that nutrition can have. They either ignore it completely, or treat it as an incredibly restrictive regime that you have to follow perfectly in order to get results. Neither is true. Anyone can make small improvements to their nutrition and reap the benefits.

Yet there's a lot of harmful messaging out there when it comes to food. You may have heard that 'food is fuel'. That is simply not true. Food is far more than just fuel. It's cultural. It's how we communicate. It's part of how we celebrate, how we mourn and how we cultivate community. The act of coming together around food, breaking bread, has been part of humanity since our very beginning.

That's why I like to put memories over muscle. Meaningful experiences, like time with friends and family, are much more important than how you look, how much muscle you have, or how much you weigh. At your funeral, no one will say, 'Oh, too bad they're gone, they had great abs.'

Of course, that doesn't mean you want to throw caution to the wind completely. As I've said, nutrition is a powerful way to improve your quality of life, prevent disease and illness, and help you to be around on this planet for a good, long time. Being fit, strong and capable can add a whole other dimension to your life. It can open doors to new adventures and experiences, add ease to your daily life, and extend your lifespan. Nutrition is just one more tool in your toolbox to help you do all that.

And hey, if visible abs or other aesthetic goals are on your wish-list, that's good too. You deserve to chase whatever goals are important to you. Whether you want to run a marathon, compete in powerlifting, do your first pull-up or fit into your favourite pair of jeans, good nutrition can help with that.

I want to help you achieve your goals and feel your best, while keeping things in perspective. Here are some core nutrition practices that will help you feel (and look) strong, healthy, and energetic – without taking over your entire life.

Nutrition practices

When you incorporate good nutrition into your life in a balanced, sustainable way there are no limits to how good you can feel.

My key practices for nutrition are as follows:

- Commit to things you can stick to
- Consume appropriate calories
- Eat enough protein and fibre

There's a lot of harmful messaging out there when it comes to food. You may have heard that 'food is fuel'. That is simply not true. Food is far more than just fuel. It's cultural. It's how we communicate. It's part of how we celebrate, how we mourn and how we cultivate community.

As you read, consider these things in order of importance. If you like, you might visualise them as a pyramid.

The first and most important practice is to commit to things you can stick to. If you aren't able to consistently adhere to any given nutrition practice, the whole thing falls apart. Keep your changes doable and repeatable – this is your foundation.

From there, consuming an appropriate amount of food – i.e. calories – is the second most important thing. If you are significantly overeating or undereating, it doesn't really matter *what* you're eating, you're probably not going to feel your best. Furthermore, if you want to get leaner, lose fat and/or gain muscle, making adjustments to your energy balance through your intake (eating less or more, according to your goals) is essential.

If you're able to strike the right energy balance, then you can consider what foods to eat. This is where protein and fibre come in. If you're going to pay attention to one food or macronutrient, pay attention to the protein! It's remarkably effective in supporting both fat loss and muscle gain, increased energy, satiation and fullness, and general health. I'll explain more about this in a moment.

At the same time, fibre matters too. Your parents were right: you do need to eat your fruit and veggies! Beans, legumes and whole grains are good too. More on this in a bit.

Again, the trick here is to commit to things you can stick to. Small, sustainable improvements in any of these areas will be far more effective than short-term, radical changes – especially over the long haul.

Eat
protein
and fibre

Consume
appropriate calories

Commit
to things you can stick to

Let's take a look at each of these practices, one by one.

Practice: Commit to things you can stick to

When people decide to improve their diet, the number one mistake they make is declaring all the things they're going to stop eating.

They say things like, 'I want to eat healthier, so I'm going to cut this food, this food and this food.'

The foods on the naughty list are usually things like sugar, bread and chocolate. In response, I tend to ask questions like: *How long do you think you can stick to that plan? How do you think it will feel to live entirely without chocolate, sugar or bread six months from now? A year from now? Are you never going to eat those foods again?*

I aim to provide a bit of a reality check because overcommitting tends to backfire. The bodybuilders I referred to previously are a perfect example: periods of high restriction are typically followed by periods of 'anything goes'. This creates a vicious cycle of restrict–binge eating patterns. The more you do this, the more it will become ingrained, and the harder it will be to change. That's why you're better off establishing long-lasting habits that will help you eat well and still enjoy your life.

Make a smart bet

As I've said before, when you take on a new habit or practice, you're essentially betting on yourself, and I want you to win that bet. So, before committing to anything, ask yourself: *Would I bet money that I can stick to this?*

Make no mistake, it's hard to make changes to your eating habits. People tend to bite off more than they can chew (excuse the pun). That's why it's especially important to commit to practices that you are at least 90 per cent – preferably 99 per cent – confident that you can maintain.

That goes for anything you read in this book, by the way. If you aren't 90–100 per cent confident you can do things exactly as I've outlined them, scale them down until you have near-total confidence in your ability to complete the task on a regular basis.

Aim for 7/10

We are humans, not robots. We don't want to eat the foods we're supposed to all the time. This is normal.

So, when it comes to your meals, aim for a 7/10. Not 10/10.

You can apply this concept in different ways. For example, you might allocate 70 per cent of one meal to foods you need, and 30 per cent of your meal to foods you want. Or you might say to yourself, out of ten meals, I'm going to make sure that seven of those meals will give my body just what my body needs, and three of those meals will be what I want.

Take this idea and use it in whatever way that works for you. My point is that you don't have to get things perfect, and you certainly don't have to get them perfect all of the time. There is room in a healthy diet for less-optimal foods, including things you eat purely for pleasure.

Don't be afraid to ask for help – especially if your goals are ambitious

Making any kind of lifestyle change, especially where food is concerned, can be challenging. This is where coaching can be incredibly helpful. A good coach can help you find a sustainable approach to your nutrition by providing education, accountability and support. If suitable, they can also help you improve your relationship with food.

Have ambitious goals? Coaching can be extra valuable. For example, if you're after significant weight loss, especially in a short span of time, a good coach can help ensure you stay safe and healthy in the process. The standard practices I'm offering in this book are useful as a general guideline, but if you want personalised programming, accountability and attention, coaching can be a great option.

To avoid getting stuck with a coach like the 'steak and nuts meal plan' guy I mentioned earlier, always be sure to ask your coach questions on why you are doing certain things. I always explain to my clients why they are doing what they are doing and why it aligns with their goals.

Practice: Consume appropriate calories

Calories are king. When it comes right down to it, *how much* you eat is more important than exactly *what* you eat – especially when it comes to body-composition goals, like fat loss or muscle gain.

Most people don't have an accurate sense of how much they're consuming, nor do they have a clear understanding of what level of intake is appropriate for their body and their goals.

Fortunately, this is really simple to figure out. There are plenty of calculators out there to help you assess your calorie target. But if you did want to do the maths yourself, the most accurate method is said to be the Mifflin-St Jeor Equation. This will help you to calculate how many calories you need to maintain your current weight; from there you can adjust the number according to your goals. (See the sidebar for more details.)

Once you know how many calories to strive for, it's a matter of hitting that target. Here are some methods to help you get a bullseye.

How to calculate your caloric needs for maintenance

Here's a quick calculation you can do to approximate your daily caloric needs, using the Mifflin-St Jeor Equation.

Step 1: Determine your BMR (Basal Metabolic Rate – the number of calories you burn as your body performs basic functions to say alive)

Females: (10 x weight in kg) + (6.25 x height in cm) – (5.0 x age in years) – 161

Males: (10 x weight in kg) + (6.25 x height in cm) – (5.0 x age in years) + 5

Step 2: Multiply the BMR by the appropriate activity factor

Sedentary – BMR × 1.2 (little to no exercise*)

Light Activity – BMR × 1.375 (light exercise 1 to 3 days per week)

Moderate Activity – BMR × 1.55 (moderate exercise 3 to 5 days per week)

Very Active – BMR × 1.725 (hard exercise 6 to 7 days per week)

Extra Active – BMR × 1.9 (very hard exercise 2 times per day, and/or a very physically demanding job)

The number you get after performing this calculation represents the approximate number of calories you would need each day to maintain your weight.

* Exercise refers to structured or planned physical activity, such as playing sports or working out. I'll explore the difference between exercise and movement, and the benefits of both, later in the book.

Track what you eat

If you don't already track your food, here's what I want you to do: for four weeks, make a note of every single thing you eat and drink.

If the idea of this gives you a headache, I get it. Tracking can be annoying at first. But you don't have to do it for ever. Four weeks is usually plenty to get into the habit of tracking and to collect adequate data. And I promise it's worth doing! As I've said, if you're not assessing, you're just guessing. Tracking your intake can give you a much better idea of how many calories you're consuming. Plus, it can help you identify what's working, and what isn't. For example, you might find some extra calories are sneaking in that you didn't realise, like mindless munching at your desk in the afternoon. Even if you decide not to change a thing, you'll still have a better understanding of yourself and your habits.

To track your food, you can use an app (like MyFitnessPal), a spreadsheet or simply go with the good old reliable pen and paper. Alternatively, you can take pictures of your meals and keep them in an album on your phone so they're easy to review.

It can be tricky to remember to track your calories. Don't beat yourself up if you forget. I've been taking tablets (digestive enzymes) at every meal for my entire life and I still forget to take them sometimes. Forgetting to do something – especially something new – is normal.

With that, here are a few tips to help you remember to track:

- Use your phone. Set alarms to remind you to track your food, at whatever times you typically eat.
- Write it down. Put a Post-it note or similar reminder on your fridge, at your desk, on the door of the snack cupboard . . . wherever you're likely to see it, especially in places that typically correspond with meal times.
- Wear a bracelet or ring. Every time you see the bracelet or ring, use it as reminder to check whether you've been tracking your calories that day. If you've forgotten, add whatever meals you've missed to your tracker, and move on.

When tracking, keep in mind that you're practising a new skill. Despite your best efforts, you might forget, fall out of the habit for a while, or miss some details. That's why I encourage you to track for a full four weeks. Consider the first two weeks a practice period; the following two weeks you're likely to be more consistent and more detailed as you get the hang of things.

Our bodies don't have opening and closing hours, therefore it's what we do on average that ultimately dictates our results. Look for the average: that's the number that will help you truly understand whether you are on track to achieve your goals, or if more adjustment is required.

To calculate your average calorie intake, add up all the calories you eat in a week (Monday–Sunday). Then divide that number by seven, which will give you your average daily calorie consumption.

Here's an example:

Monday (2,312)

Tuesday (1,567)

Wednesday (2,301)

Thursday (1,785)

Friday (2,156)

Saturday (3,100)

Sunday (1,745)

Total: 14,966

Average: 14,966 ÷ 7 = 2,138 calories

Make incremental changes

Once you've assessed how many calories you need per day to achieve your goal and you've tracked your intake for a few weeks, you may find there is a significant difference between how many calories you typically eat and how many you need to eat.

For example, suppose you need to eat 1,800 calories per day in order to lose weight. After tracking your eating habits, you realise you typically eat 2,500 calories a day.

> *Our bodies don't have opening and closing hours, therefore it's what we do on average that ultimately dictates our results.*

If this is the case, I wouldn't recommend you drop right down to 1,800, unless you're working with a trusted coach.

Instead, I would encourage you to eat 250 fewer calories each day for two or three weeks. (So, using this example, you'd start eating 2,250 calories a day.) Once you're comfortable with this reduction, you could drop down another 250 and aim for 2,000 calories per day. After two or three more weeks, you could drop down by another 200 and make 1,800 calories a day your target. By doing this in incremental stages, you'll become acclimatised to the changes and it won't feel like such a shock.

This goes for calorie increases too. Smaller changes over time will help you adjust so the changes don't feel as radical.

Aim for the average

As mentioned, it's how much you eat on average – not daily – that matters. We're humans, not robots. We shouldn't expect ourselves to eat a precise amount of food every single day. The trick is to consume appropriate calories on average, throughout the course of a week. Ideally, by the end of the week, your calories will roughly add up to the number you want to hit.

By aiming for the average, you don't have to worry about getting things exactly right every single day. Some days you might eat a bit more, and other days you might eat a bit less. If it averages out to roughly the amount you're aiming for by the end of the week, you're golden.

Here's an added tip for this, especially if you work Monday to Friday and want to enjoy some more flexibility on weekends. Focus on keeping your eating habits structured and consistent during the week. (Planning your meals in advance can help; there are some more tips and shortcuts for this below.) If you eat a bit less than you need on weekdays, you can 'bank' some extra calories for the weekend. By keeping your calories lower on regular days, you'll have more freedom to enjoy movie nights, birthdays, dinners

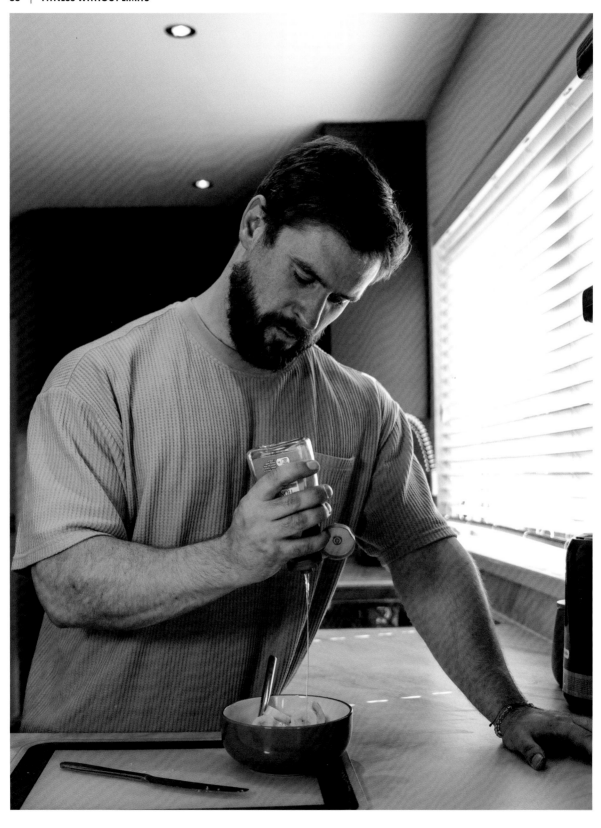

with friends and so on – without blowing past your calorie requirements. This allows you to enjoy your time off without feeling like you're restricting yourself. Another bonus is you can look forward to and savour these meals even more than you normally would.

Break your calorie requirements into meals

Now that you have your calorie targets established, here's a simple trick to meet those targets without constantly having to do maths.

Once you've worked out your daily calorie requirements, split that figure into three meals.

For example, if your goal is to eat 2,500 calories a day, each meal might contain roughly 800 calories. Or breakfast might contain 600 calories, lunch 800 calories, and dinner 1,100. You can split the calories up depending on how you like to eat.

Now that you know your calorie goals, come up with some options for yourself. I like to have two standard options for each meal that meet my calorie requirements. Obviously, you don't have to eat these same meals over and over again, but having a couple of 'go-to' options can make things easy.

If you're a busy person, try to come up with at least one option for each meal that is quick and convenient for you to prepare. For example, one of my go-to lunches is a can of tuna, some microwaved rice and a salad, with a little sweet chili sauce for spice. This meal fits my calorie requirements and it's very easy to prepare, so it works well on my busiest days.

If you get bored with the options you create for yourself, go back to the drawing board and come up with some more possibilities. Mix and match as you plan your weekly menus.

Eating appropriate calories: a tale of two clients

What exactly do I mean when I say, 'eat appropriate calories'? Depending on various factors – including your starting point, your needs, goals, body type and existing habits – the answer will be different. For some people, this means scaling up their energy intake (i.e. eating more) and for some, it means scaling down (i.e. eating less).

Let's take a look at two of my clients. Christos and Siobhan had similar goals: they both wanted to lose weight. But their situations – and the exact methods I used to help them achieve their goals – were different.

Christos came to me shortly before his thirtieth birthday. He wanted to enter his thirties feeling and looking more fit. His specific goals were to feel confident enough to take his shirt off at the beach, and be able to keep up with his friends when cycling. To maintain his weight of 77 kilos (170 lbs), Christos needed to eat about 2,500 calories a day, but he had become accustomed to consuming around 2,800 calories per day.

For Christos to achieve his goals, he needed to eat fewer calories than he was burning. Under my careful supervision, we decided to go for an aggressive deficit. Christos dropped his daily calorie intake down to 2,000 calories per day, while making protein the focus of his meals. I checked in with him regularly about his energy levels, strength and recovery, and he assured me that he was feeling good, exercising well, and recovering quickly after his workouts.

With this strategy, Christos lost 4 kilos (about 9 lbs) in eleven weeks. He also gained confidence and improved his cycling times.

Here's where I'd like to give you the 'don't try this at home,' warning. I don't recommend dropping to a severe calorie deficit on your own; if you want to try a strategy like this, work with a coach who can ensure you stay safe and healthy in the process.

Now let's consider Siobhan. Siobhan was in her early forties and extremely busy. A mother of three young children, including a child who has cystic fibrosis, Siobhan was so busy looking after everyone else that she rarely considered her own needs. As a result, she was eating very little, about 1,300 calories a day, and her nutritional quality wasn't great. At 77 kilos (170 lbs), Siobhan wanted to lose weight – so she assumed she'd have to cut her calories even lower. Instead, we did something different: I encouraged her to increase her calorie intake slightly, while adding in more protein. My intention was to give Siobhan more energy, so she could move around more, thereby burning more calories *and* giving her body adequate nutrition.

In addition to having more energy, increasing protein also adds to the thermic effect of food. In layperson terms, the thermic effect of food refers to how hard your body has to work – how many calories it has to burn – to digest your food. Some foods, like protein, require more work from your digestive system, meaning your body has to burn more calories to digest them. When you eat more protein, you burn more calories. A nice little bonus!

With my guidance, Siobhan bumped up both her protein and calorie intake, aiming for 1,400–1,500 calories per day. This is still a low-calorie diet, but remember, it was an increase from where she started. I always work with the individual in front of me and take their starting point into consideration.

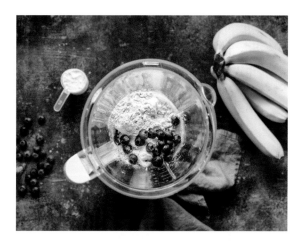

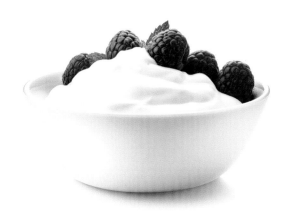

To help Siobhan do this, we focused on adding some high-protein snacks. She typically didn't have much time for sit-down meals and her energy tended to lag in the middle of the day. So, we came up with two quick snacks containing protein: one was Greek yoghurt with a handful of raspberries on top; the other was a protein shake that she could whip up in two minutes by tossing a scoop of protein powder, a banana and some ice into a blender. This simple change gave Siobhan more energy throughout

the day. Her movement and step count throughout the day naturally increased.

With this approach, Siobhan lost 18.5 kilos (41 lbs) in twenty-four weeks.

As you can see, Christos and Siobhan are two different people, who used two different strategies. But both lost weight without sacrificing energy or strength.

You may also notice that while the exact strategies were different – one person consumed fewer calories, the other person consumed more – the core principles were quite similar: both clients focused on eating appropriate calories and consuming adequate protein.

Practice: **Eat enough protein and fibre**

When it comes to what you eat, the two main things to concentrate on are protein and fibre. That's right: you don't need to worry about your carbs, fats, micronutrients, supplements or anything else you can dream up.

Unless you're an elite athlete or have a specific health condition, protein and fibre are the only two food groups that you need to focus on. That's because these are, far and away, going to give you the best results for the least amount of effort. On the other hand, if you start to make your meals more complicated than this, you'll wind up putting yourself in some sort of nutritional prison, and there's no reason for that. The fact is, if you concentrate on adequate protein and adequate fibre, you'll have what you need for a lean, strong, healthy body.

Eat more protein

While protein has many roles in the body, it is vital for muscle growth, as it helps to repair and maintain muscle tissue. If we don't have the amount our body needs, we will not be able to fully recover from our workouts or the wear-and-tear of daily life. Protein is also useful for weight loss as it will make you feel fuller for longer, keeping your body satisfied and reducing your appetite. A lack of sufficient protein may cause you to feel weak and hungry, as protein is an important source of energy. It can also affect your immune system, increasing your chance of getting sick and making recovery from illness take longer. You get the message: eat more protein!

So, how much protein should you eat? The general rule to go by is 1 gram of protein per pound of bodyweight per day. So, if you weigh 150 lbs (or 68 kilos) you'd aim to eat 150 grams of protein each day. However, this isn't a hard and fast rule, and you have to go with what is both realistic and manageable for you. Depending on how much protein you currently eat, this may sound like a lot, so here's a simple trick. Every time you plan a meal, start with the protein, then work everything else around it. Consider the protein the focus of the meal and everything else as an accompaniment.

Keep things interesting for yourself. We all know a plain chicken breast isn't overly exciting, but you can mix things up by trying new herbs and spices. There

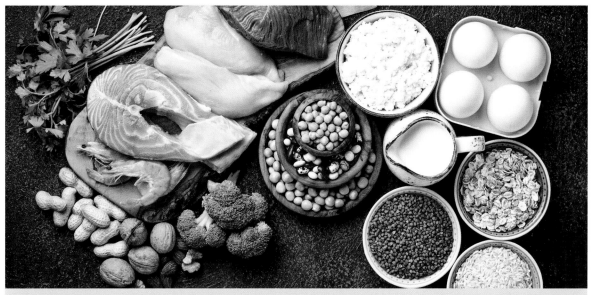

Good sources of protein include:

- ▶ Lean beef
- ▶ Chicken
- ▶ Turkey
- ▶ Salmon
- ▶ Prawns
- ▶ Eggs
- ▶ Cottage cheese
- ▶ Beans and legumes, such as lentils and chickpeas
- ▶ Quinoa
- ▶ Tofu
- ▶ Greek yoghurt
- ▶ Protein powder

are plenty of flavour sachets available in shops these days. You can also challenge yourself to try out proteins you're less familiar with – speak to your butcher or fishmonger for some inspiration, or trade recipes with adventurous friends.

Eat more fibre

Just like protein, fibre has loads of benefits. It supports gut health, helps stabilise blood glucose levels, lowers cholesterol levels and improves bowel health . . . just to list a few. As a bonus, fibre-rich foods are typically high in micronutrients such as vitamin C, magnesium and zinc, which support recovery.

General recommendations for fibre intake are 30–38 grams of fibre per day for the average male, 21–25 grams per day for the average female. Admittedly, fruits and vegetables can be tricky to track. You don't need to be weighing spinach leaves – who's got time for all that? To ensure you're getting enough, aim to have a hand-sized amount of fibrous foods with each meal.

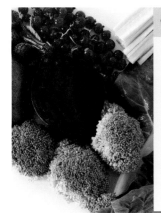

Good sources of fibre include:

▶ Broccoli	▶ Pears
▶ Carrots	▶ Kiwis
▶ Beetroot	▶ Raspberries and blackberries
▶ Baby spinach	▶ Beans and legumes
▶ Artichokes	▶ Chia seeds
▶ Avocado	▶ Wholegrains
▶ Apples	▶ Popcorn

If you're familiar with macronutrients, you might notice that fibrous foods are also carbohydrates. While that's true, I prefer to focus on consuming fibre rather than carbs in general. It can be easy to consume carbohydrates without getting adequate fibre; for example, you could get eat a load of chips, sweets and white bread, and you'd get all the carbs you need. But your body would be lacking in fibre – not to mention all the other great nutrients that fibrous foods tend to provide. When you focus on fibre, you ensure that you give your body what it needs, and your carbohydrate requirements will naturally be taken care of without intentional effort. I'll explain a bit more about macronutrients shortly.

Use shortcuts

One of the biggest challenges people face is running out of time to plan and cook their meals. I always advise clients not to be afraid to take shortcuts. The more you can minimise potential roadblocks, guesswork and energy, the more likely you'll be to stick to your plan.

Here are some tricks I use:

- Buy pre-cut and/or pre-cooked food. For example, many grocery stores sell pre-cut vegetables; some stores even have 'stir fry' or 'roast' mixes where vegetables are all cut up and ready to go. I also like to buy pre-cooked, pre-cut chicken breast strips. That way, all I have to do is add them to my wraps at lunch.

- Meal delivery or meal-prep services. If you can afford it, such services can be useful, especially during very busy periods. My wife and I subscribe to a meal-prep service where the food arrives pre-measured and pre-portioned. This takes the mental energy out of planning and shopping, and it makes cooking dinner quick and painless.
- For a quick protein boost, make a protein shake. You can even make it the night before, throw it into a jar or shaker bottle, and give it a quick shake in the morning. I like mine with a scoop of whey protein powder, a spoonful of almond butter, a handful of blueberries, and a scoop of oats, but yours can be even simpler. Ideally, you'll get most of your protein from whole food sources, but supplementing with a protein powder can be really useful, especially when you're short on time.

Eat the rainbow

As much as possible, aim to eat a variety of foods, including a range of colourful fruits and vegetables. This will boost your fibre intake and as a bonus it will give you a range of micronutrients (vitamins and minerals) to support good health.

To practise eating the rainbow, one of my clients came up with a great idea. He made a checklist of all the fruits and vegetables he enjoys, laminated it and hung it on his fridge. Every week, he looks at the list. Each time he eats one of the foods, he ticks it off the list using a dry erase marker. Throughout the week, he can see the array of veggies he's eaten.

This fun little practice encourages him to eat a diverse mix of fruit and veg each week. I love this because it's a way of gamifying something that could otherwise feel boring or complicated. Feel free to steal this idea!

Drink water

Good hydration is always a good thing, but it's especially important to be conscious of your water intake when consuming fibre. Otherwise, you could wind up feeling bloated and constipated. You'll want to drink at least 2–3 litres of water per day. The bigger you are (both in height and mass), the more you need to drink. Ditto if you sweat a lot.

What about macros?

You may have heard some buzz about macronutrients, or 'macros', and if you use an app like MyFitnessPal, you might be wondering if you need to count your macros along with your calories.

If you're unfamiliar with macros, here's a quick overview. Macronutrients are a group of nutrients that the body needs. The three essential macronutrients are protein, carbohydrates and fat.

Each of these macronutrients are important for good health. I've already covered the benefits of protein; of the three macronutrients, protein is hands-down the most important one, especially when it comes to maintaining a healthy body composition, gaining muscle mass and/or losing fat.

The other two are also important, though, so I'll cover them briefly here.

Let's begin with carbohydrates. Carbohydrates serve as the primary source of energy for our cells. They come in various forms, including sugars, starches and fibres. In the body, carbohydrates play several notable roles. For one thing, carbohydrates are the body's preferred and most readily available source of energy. When consumed, they are broken down into glucose, which is absorbed into the bloodstream and transported to cells to be used as fuel for various metabolic processes. Glucose derived from these carbohydrates is important for brain function. The brain relies heavily on glucose as its primary energy source, and a steady supply of carbohydrates is necessary to maintain cognitive function and support overall mental wellbeing.

Here's another useful thing to keep in mind, especially if you're ever contemplated a low-carb diet. When we have an adequate carbohydrate intake, we spare proteins from being used as an energy source. That's because when carbohydrates are insufficient, the body may break down proteins from muscles and other tissues to produce glucose through a process called gluconeogenesis. In other words: don't cut out carbs completely, or your body will steal away your precious muscle mass and use it for energy!

Despite the benefits of carbohydrates, as I mentioned earlier, I think it's better to zoom in a bit and put your focus on consuming fibre rather than tracking carbs in general.

Now let's consider fat. While it's been vilified at times, especially during the 'low-fat diet' trend popularised in the nineties, dietary fat plays a valuable role in a healthy diet. Among other things, fat provides energy, supports cell function, and may even help reduce the risk of age-related diseases. Fat is vital for producing essential fatty acids, which are building blocks for hormones and other crucial molecules in the body. That said, fat is also higher in energy (calories) and it's best not to over-consume it. Unless you're on a low-fat diet – which I don't recommend unless you have a specific health issue – you'll probably consume adequate fats through your natural eating habits without having to count your macros. That said, some fat sources are definitely better than others. When possible, aim to avoid trans fats, oxidised fats and hydrogenated fats. Keep highly processed foods, fried foods and saturated vegetable oils to a minimum. Instead, look for whole-food sources of fat such as fatty fish, extra virgin olive oil, avocado, whole eggs, nuts and seeds.

If macros are important, shouldn't I track them?

Hopefully, you can start to see why I emphasise eating protein and fibre – while also eating appropriate calories – as nutritional priorities. Here's some additional food for thought as to why I don't recommend counting your macros.

My biggest issue with macro counting is that it starts to be extremely limiting. Trying to get an exact quantity of protein, fats and carbs in each meal can become a complex juggling act. For example, suppose you planned to have chicken breast with green beans for dinner. Depending on the macros you're trying to reach, this meal might be too low in carbs, so let's say you add in some rice. And then you realise there's not enough fat in your chicken breast to meet your fat macro, so you swap that out for salmon. These adjustments increase the overall calorie intake of your meal, so now you must figure out what not to eat to stay within your daily calorie quota. You're now working on re-configuring your entire meal, which was perfectly fine to begin with. And that's a meal at home; forget trying to go out for dinner and

enjoy a fun evening with friends! As I said earlier, I'm want you to be able to live a full and healthy life with as few restrictions as possible. Macro counting creates unnecessary complications and limitations.

Here's an alternative idea to work with. Think about your meals like a glass of water.

The top of the glass represents your ideal calorie intake. You don't want to overflow the glass, but you'd like to fill it somewhere near the top.

Now imagine the glass is already 25 per cent full. That's your minimum amount of protein.

Beyond that 25 per cent, you can fill the glass up however else you like. Want to fill 25 per cent of your glass with protein, 50 per cent with carbs and 25 per cent with fat? Fine. Or how about 60 per cent protein, 30 per cent carbs and 10 per cent fat? No problem. Or 40 per cent protein, 40 per cent carbs and 20 per cent fat. All good – as long as the totals don't overflow your glass.

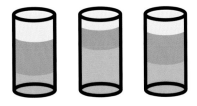

My point is that as long as you're getting adequate protein and sticking to your calorie requirements, the rest of the exact calculations aren't particularly important. (Although, as you know, I do recommend you eat fibre. For the sake of this analogy, you can consider carbs and fibre interchangeable.)

If you're unsure of whether you're drinking enough, sneak a peek at your urine. I tell my clients, 'If your pee is yellow, drink more my fellow. If your pee is clear, you're in the clear.'

If you're not used to drinking water, it can take time to build the habit. I recommend getting a reusable bottle (avoid plastic for the sake of the environment, please) and keep it handy. Place it on your desk while you're at work, or stick it in the cup-holder of your car if you're driving for long periods of time. This will serve as a visual reminder to keep drinking.

No foods are 'off-limits'

You may have noticed that I've encouraged you to eat *more* of certain foods. (And, when discussing fats and carbs, less of others.) But I have yet to tell you that a single food is off-limits entirely.

I do that deliberately, because the point of the 'fitness without limits' approach is that nothing is off-limits. We're trying to create fewer limits in our lives, not more. I like to tell my clients that the goal is to have as much fun and flexibility as they can get away with. There's no need to trap yourself into following a restrictive diet or remove certain foods (or entire food groups or macronutrients) from your diet altogether.

If you're used to thinking that certain foods are bad ('sugar is poison' or 'carbs make you fat'), here's a little concept to keep in mind: the danger is in the dosage. Almost anything can be toxic given the right quantity. Even water – something that is essential for life. Go without water for long and you'll die. But it is possible to die from excessive water intake in extreme (and highly unusual) circumstances. Yet we don't say that water is bad for you. The same goes for just about anything.

Give your body what it needs, while also giving yourself what *you* need. Take your holiday. Go out with your friends. Improving your nutrition shouldn't mean you put your life on hold. There are almost always ways to make small improvements without imposing lots of restrictions on yourself. In the end, my goal is for you to have the most unlimited life possible. Good nutrition is just another tool to help you do that.

Summary

If we're lucky enough to have access to it, food should not be stressful. Food rules can easily become a prison, if we let them. But there's no need for that.

Good nutrition can be far simpler than it's made out to be. Eat an appropriate amount for your goals. Eat enough protein. Eat enough fibre. It's as simple as that.

Admittedly, changing your eating habits can be uncomfortable. (I still wrestle with making eggs in the morning when I'd much rather pour myself a bowl of cereal.) Be nice to yourself as you work towards incremental improvements, and don't stress if you slip up. If you keep working towards your goal at a steady and sustainable pace, you will make progress.

Most importantly, avoid the trap of taking too much on at once, or committing to some kind of diet or programme you can't (and probably shouldn't) stick to. Keep your changes small and simple and you'll get better results over time – I promise. And if you need help keeping things in perspective, remember the mantra: *memories over muscle*.

 RECAP

Your key nutrition practices are:

- Commit to things you can stick to
- Consume appropriate calories
- Eat enough protein and fibre

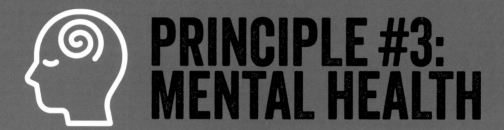

PRINCIPLE #3: MENTAL HEALTH

've had people describe me as 'relentlessly optimistic'. I'm not a ray of sunshine all the time, but I do tend to have a good attitude and an enthusiastic outlook. You'll rarely find me stewing in a bad mood for long.

There's a reason for that.

Growing up with cystic fibrosis, I often felt as though there were two versions of me. There's the 'real me', and then there's the dark, evil version that has CF. The CF version is like the Terminator: it's relentless. It wants to chase me, and it will not stop. It never takes a break; it just keeps coming.

As I've said, building my strength and maintaining markers of good health have helped put some distance between me and the feeling that the 'CF Terminator' is just around the corner. But the fear of it returning keeps me on edge. In my darker moments, my entire life feels fragile. My evil inner voice tells me, *You could be one just infection away from being in hospital again.* All my plans, hopes and dreams for the future feel precarious, like they could fall apart at any moment.

I've also known a lot of people who have passed away. Some of their lives were tragically short. (This is in part because of my connection with the CF community, though not entirely. I'll tell you more about one person in particular a bit later in this section.) My experience watching others lose their

> **As much as possible, I want to live with appreciation and contentment, and use my time here to help others.**

lives has given me an even sharper awareness that life is precious. Living with such awareness can be a double-edged sword. On the one hand, it can encourage you to make the most of every day. But it can also send you into a spiral. Some people with CF choose to be reckless with their lives and their health; they fall into traps such as alcoholism and drug use, because they don't believe they have much of a future to fight for. It's probably obvious that I choose the former: as much as possible, I want to live with appreciation and contentment, and use my time here to help others.

I have come to accept that I can't out-fitness my inner Terminator. Yes, getting bigger and stronger did ease some of my fears, but it didn't make them go away completely. Eventually I realised that I could either spend my entire life trying to get bigger, faster and stronger in the hope that my deep, dark fears would go away completely, or I could learn some mental strategies and practices to prevent my limitations – or perceived limitations – from controlling my entire life. Clearly, I went with option B. I've made caring for my mind just as much a part of my life as caring for my body. This approach has allowed me to move forward with my life from a place of ease and lightness. (For the most part, anyway – I'm only human.) Just as I see fitness not as a luxury but a necessity in my life, my mental health is non-negotiable, and it requires regular, deliberate effort.

My experiences are not unique, of course. I have no doubt you have your own version of the kinds of challenges I've described. We all carry with us a unique mix of self-limiting beliefs, assumptions about what we can't do, fears about our future and doubts about our potential.

Furthermore, we all have a unique make-up that influences our mental health and wellness; some individuals have mental health conditions that make life harder. There are many things we don't have control over. But if we let these things rule us, we'll miss out on the richness that life has to offer.

Fortunately, there are aspects of mental health that we can, if not entirely control, at least have influence over. We can choose to practise a positive mindset that will help us better navigate the ups and downs of life. We can choose to use techniques that support a good mood, even on our worst days. And, importantly, we can choose to appreciate ourselves and our lives rather than focusing on our limitations.

Working regularly on my own mental health has taught me that it is possible to create a pleasant mental space for yourself, but it does take work. It's a bit like cleaning your house: you have to keep at it. Clean your home once and it looks great, but if you ignore it for a few weeks, the dirty dishes will pile up, the shelves will get dusty, and soon it won't be a very nice place to live. Your mental health is the same: it requires regular attention.

Physical health is nothing without mental health

If you're relentlessly chasing your ideal body, and think mental health is just 'fluffy stuff', consider this some tough love.

In a society that puts so much emphasis on physical appearance, it's no wonder that people tend to focus on aesthetic goals such as fat loss or muscle gain. I'm more than happy to help clients with these kinds of goals. But I also notice that many people approach these goals thinking (subconsciously or not), *When I achieve my goal*, then *I'll be happy*. It can be tempting to assume that any mental health stuff you're wrestling with, including self-criticism and body image issues, will naturally improve and everything fall into place once you've achieved your goal. But this is a fallacy.

If you neglect your mental health, it will not matter how much you can bench press, how many burpees you can do, or how good you look in a bathing suit – you will still be unhappy. In fact, you might even feel worse when you achieve your goal because it will be painfully clear that it was not the magic bullet you were hoping for. Trust me: I've known people who look the fittest a person can look, who can perform at the peak of their game, and otherwise represent the pinnacle of human health, who are nonetheless completely miserable.

The reality is, if you aren't in a position to appreciate what you've got, it doesn't matter how fit you are, how good you look, how well you can perform or how 'healthy' you are. I learned this first-hand when I was the healthiest I'd ever been and yet had become so self-critical and concerned with my appearance that I couldn't relax and enjoy it.

So much of life is perception. Your perception will dictate your progress. And perception is a fickle thing. Have you ever woken up one morning, looked in the mirror and been absolutely convinced you've gained weight and turned soft overnight? Your mood and mental state can dramatically influence how you feel about yourself and how you interpret your progress. I've had clients who absolutely smash their goals – lose the weight, and lose it quickly – yet still crumble to pieces because their mental state causes them to perceive everything through a negative, self-critical lens. For better or worse, progress is in the mind.

Beyond that, the worse your mental state, the harder it is to get yourself to keep going. Many people have become far too good at beating themselves up, thinking that speaking harshly to themselves will inspire them to be better. But human beings don't work that way. Being nasty to yourself only puts additional obstacles in your way. Motivation and self-discipline are much harder to muster if you feel bad.

The good news, of course, is that when you attend to your mental health, everything gets better. It's easier to get back up and try again if you have a positive outlook. It's more fun to work towards goals and solve challenges when you're in a good mood. And when you can challenge your internalised assumptions about your own limitations, you learn that you have more potential than you ever realised – and that is a very fun thing to discover.

It comes down to this: the more you tend to your inner state of being, the easier everything else gets. The best part is, no matter your starting point, mental wellbeing is something you can practise and improve upon – just like any other aspect of fitness.

A great example of this is my client Jenny. When Jenny started training with me, all she could see were what she considered to be her faults. She was reluctant to go to the gym because she didn't want to be seen by other people, and when she did eventually go, she felt extremely self-conscious. Even in the height of summer (an Irish summer, but summer nonetheless) she wore a big hoodie the entire time to cover herself up.

> ## The more you tend to your inner state of being, the easier everything else gets.

I wanted to help Jenny build her confidence, so we started by setting reasonable, achievable goals. I knew Jenny would beat herself up if she missed a workout, so we made sure her expectations were reasonable.

Throughout our work together, I noticed a pattern. Jenny tended to focus on what she perceived as signs of failure or mistakes, rather than keeping an eye on the big picture. I encouraged her to continually look back to where she had started so she could see the progress she'd made. For example, while the scale might not move every single week, she could review old photos and clearly see that she'd lost weight. And while she might not reach her desired step-count every day, I reminded her that on average, she was walking far more than she used to. At the same time, I encouraged Jenny to practise some self-compassion and to appreciate the effort she was putting in, even if she wasn't always making as much progress as she wished.

We also worked on Jenny's tendency to compare herself to others, particularly fitness models on Instagram. I shared a bit of behind-the-scenes info on that, reminding Jenny that many of the people she admired live unhealthy lifestyles involving restrict–binge cycles. At my recommendation, Jenny stopped following people who triggered her body image issues, and started seeking out content that emphasises self-kindness and celebrates various body types.

Over time, with more perspective and self-compassion, Jenny's confidence increased. Eventually, the hoodie came off. She even reduced her antidepressant medication. Over the course of twenty-four weeks, Jenny lost nearly 14 kilos (30 lbs). As I write this, she's lost nearly 10 per cent of her starting bodyweight.

Six months after we started working together, Jenny sent me a picture of herself and her wife at Disneyland. She was holding up Thor's hammer while wearing a sleeveless top. Jenny beamed at the camera, emanating ease and joy. I teared up when I saw the photo, because I knew it represented an incredible inner transformation for her. Jenny later said to me, 'If you'd told me earlier that I would feel this good, and this good about myself, I never would have believed you.'

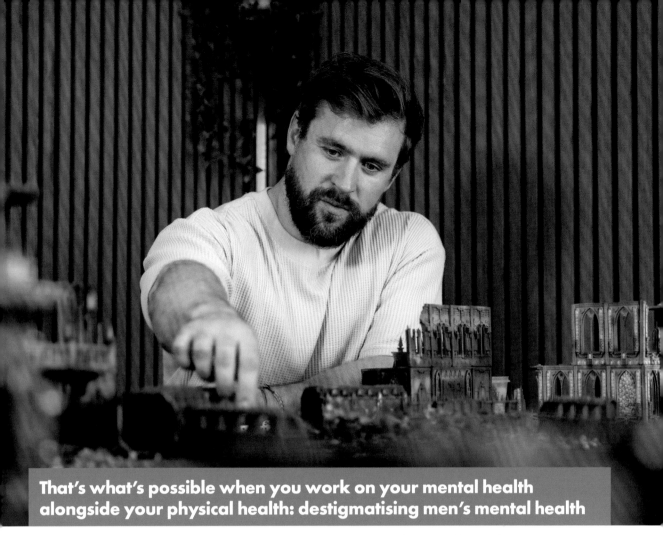

That's what's possible when you work on your mental health alongside your physical health: destigmatising men's mental health

I first saw *The Lord of the Rings* when I was about twelve. The film had an impact on me in a number of ways (it's the reason I wanted to become a director), but one of its impacts has only recently surfaced for me.

During my annual re-watch, I noticed that throughout the movie, men cry. They console each other. A particular scene that stands out for me is (spoiler alert!) after Gandalf seemingly dies in the mines of Moria. Here, we see the impact on the entire fellowship: the men break down in tears, having to comfort one another. This is one of many scenes in the trilogy where men openly cry when experiencing pain and sorrow.

It's ridiculous to me that so many men are still taught that it's not okay to cry. Crying goes hand-in-hand with laughter; if you tell men not to cry, you might as well tell them not to laugh, either. Crying and laughter are just different points on the emotional spectrum that all humans, regardless of sex or gender, are born with.

Expressing your emotions and sharing your feelings with people you trust is an important part of mental health. And not just painful emotions, but love and joy too. A few years ago, I started saying 'I love you' to my closest friends at the end of every phone call. It's reciprocal; they say it back. It might seem unusual for two men in a platonic relationship to say I love you to each other, but we need to change that. We all need to feel loved and appreciated.

Mental health practices

There are plenty of mental health practices out there, and the list you're about to read is by no means exhaustive. Part of good mental health is discovering which practices and habits work best for you.

My number-one recommendation is to try things. If you're reluctant to try one of my suggestions here, my advice is to give it a go it anyway. If it doesn't seem to help, you don't have to keep doing it. But if you don't try, you'll never know. Caring for your mental health is an ongoing practice of self-exploration, so the best thing you can do is simply get started.

With that in my mind, my key practices for mental health are as follows:

- Breathe
- Foster appreciation
- Cultivate meaningful relationships

Practice: **Breathe**

Take a moment right now and pay attention to your breath. What do you notice? Can you feel yourself breathing?

Breath is vital to life. It's something we have complete control over, yet it can become passive. We forget we're even doing it. By shifting our attention towards our breath, we ground ourselves in the present. Paying attention to your breathing can pull you out of whatever is happening in your imagination and re-focus you into the now.

Conscious, deep breathing can also engage the parasympathetic nervous system, which means it helps your body relax. If you're anxious, panicky, stressed or in a 'fight or flight' state, slow breathing can help your body calm down. It sends a message to your body that you're safe and everything is okay. Thus, while deliberate breathing can be useful at any time, it can be especially useful in times of stress. It's also a handy technique to try when going to sleep at night.

In addition to the stress-relieving benefits, I'd also encourage you to focus on your breathing because it's something we tend to take for granted.

Not everyone has the luxury of breathing easily and naturally. Remember how lucky you are to breathe; focusing on this can help you shift out of anxiety or stress and into a more appreciative state. More on the benefits of appreciation in a moment.

Box breathing

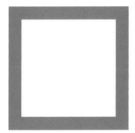

There's a technique I use frequently called box breathing. You can use this technique whenever you like, including when you feel stressed. Personally, I do this if I feel nervous, such as when I get my bloods taken. I hate needles, but this simple practice calms me down and helps me move through it.

Here's how it works. Imagine a square box. If you like, you can find a square or square-like shape somewhere within your line of sight. It doesn't have to be a perfect square, just something with a similar shape.

Step 1: starting from the bottom left corner, draw your eyes up the left-hand side of the box and inhale through your nose. Slowly count to four while inhaling as much as you can.

Step 2: moving your vision from left to right along the top of the box, hold your breath for another slow count of four.

Step 3: moving your vision down from the top to the bottom of the right-hand side of the box, exhale from your mouth and count to four again. Aim to let all the air out of your lungs.

Step 4: moving your vision from right to left along the bottom of the box, hold your breath once more, slowly counting to four once more.

Repeat the process as often as you like.

If you prefer, you can skip the visual and just conduct the breathing part of the exercise. I find the image of a box helps me relax and move through the process, but do whatever works for you. Some people find it helps to close their eyes and/or put a hand on their belly while breathing.

Practice: Foster appreciation

There was a massive turning point in my life that I haven't mentioned until now, but it's been in the back of my mind the whole time I've been writing this book, and I think this is the right time to share it with you.

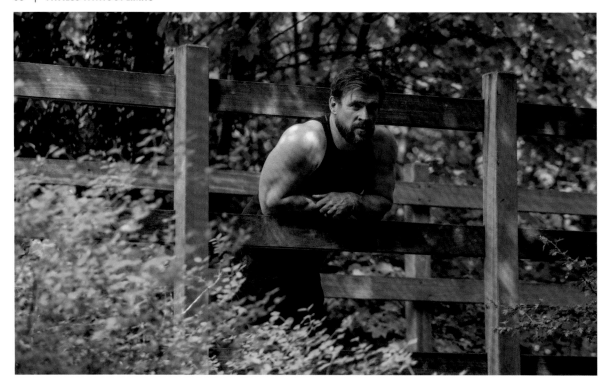

When I was seventeen years old, one of my very best friends – who was the same age as me – passed away. His name was Mark and he was an incredible person. He always made everyone feel comfortable in his presence. He was effortlessly cool and friendly, and loved to show off his amazing dance skills at talent shows and parties.

Mark died suddenly due to complications after a routine surgery. Losing him turned my entire world upside down. One day he was here, the next he simply . . . wasn't. I was devastated.

After Mark died, I saw the world differently. As a teenager, even one with CF, you think you're invincible. Losing Mark burst that bubble and I was forced to come to terms with the fact that none of us knows how much time we have. That whole 'life is precious' cliché? I learned at that moment just how brutally true it is.

Losing Mark is one of the reasons I became determined to get fitter and healthier. I recognised that I couldn't take my health for granted, especially with CF, and I would have to be relentlessly deliberate in my efforts to stay well.

At the same time, Mark's death cast new light on what it means to me to be alive. It made me immensely sad to think about all the life that Mark would miss out on. In turn, this made me absolutely determined not to miss out on living my own. I made a promise to myself not to take things for granted, and to truly appreciate all the good things I have in my life. For as long as I'm alive, I decided, I wanted to be the 'most alive' I can be.

By and large, I continue to uphold this promise. Appreciation has become a cornerstone of my approach to everything. In my own life, and as a coach, I've come to see how much of a game-changer the simple act of appreciation can be. After all, it's incredibly easy to focus on all the things we don't have, all the things we lack, all the things we aren't good at and all the things we dislike about ourselves or others. Self-improvement is great, but it can become a problem if it takes you away from appreciating life and sends you into a pit of self-criticism and negativity.

As I mentioned earlier, the arrival fantasy that says 'I'll be happy when . . .' is just that: a fantasy. Buying into the idea that you will only be happy once you achieve your goals prevents you from appreciating the moment you're currently in. If you delay happiness for the 'perfect' moment, you'll be waiting for ever. But if you choose to work towards your dreams and goals *while appreciating what you already have*, you can increase your potential for contentment and joy *right now*.

Happiness itself is a fantasy of sorts because it's a fleeting state. A wonderful state, sure, but not something that's going to stick around for ever. Appreciation, on the other hand, is something we can choose to experience at any point. It does not mean ignoring whatever challenges you're currently facing. Nor does it mean you have to be blissfully ignorant of things that are genuinely difficult or unpleasant in your life. And you don't have to live in a constant state of ignorance or toxic positivity. Rather, appreciation invites you to create some mental space for whatever is worth appreciating in the here and now.

Take a moment right now to try it out. Take a second and see if you can come up with three things that you appreciate about your life. This simple act has the potential to transform your mood at any time.

Conduct a daily appreciation practice

To get the maximum mental health benefits of appreciation, I recommend making the little practice I just shared with you – listing three things you appreciate – part of your daily routine.

To make this a habit, choose a time of day when you typically have a couple of minutes to yourself. At that time each day you're going to make a note of three things you appreciate. Ideally, write them down in a journal, notebook or on your phone.

Inevitably, you'll forget – it's human nature. So set reminders. For example, if you want to do this in the morning, you might stick a Post-it note on your bathroom mirror that says 'three things' on it, as a cue to remember. One of my clients has a little action figure that sits on top of his coffee maker – when he makes his coffee in the morning, the action figure reminds him to write out his three things while the coffee brews.

When you first try this practice, you might start listing the obvious. For example, you might come up with something like, 'I appreciate my kids, my health and having a roof over my head.' Those are all wonderful things to list. But after you've done this a couple of times, try to get a bit more granular. Aim to notice things that you might not have noticed – things that you might easily take for granted if you don't deliberately bring your awareness to them.

Here's one of my own. I love the smell of my dog, Ollie. When I lean into him and breathe in the scent of his fur, it calms me right down. Simply appreciating this detail makes me feel calmer. It also reminds me that there will come a time when he is no longer around and I won't get to breathe in that wonderful smell any more, so I'm further reminded to appreciate him while he's here.

Focus on what you can do (not on what you can't)

As a coach, I've come to notice that most people are hyper-aware of their limitations. Injuries, illnesses, chronic health conditions, mobility issues, scheduling restraints or even strong preferences such as 'I hate cardio' or 'I can't stand to be hungry', may seem like immovable forces in their lives.

While some limitations might be changeable (for example, injuries may heal; schedules may be adjusted; preferences may evolve), some are not. There may be actual, hard-and-fast limits on certain activities or movement in your life.

And that's okay. The trick – the skill, really – is to learn to focus on what you *can* do. Appreciate that. Celebrate that. Build on that.

It doesn't have to be physical. You can observe and appreciate things you like about yourself such as mental, social or emotional strengths.

To build this skill, extend the appreciation practice you just learned about and apply it to yourself. For example, if you're frustrated by a physical limitation, write down three things you appreciate about your body right now. How *can* you move? What *does* your body do well?

It doesn't have to be physical, either. You can observe and appreciate things you like about yourself such as mental strengths you have, social strengths or emotional strengths.

To put this into action, you have some options. If you like, you can tack this on to your existing appreciation practice, so you're listing six things in total. Or you can incorporate it into another habit, such as going to the gym or sitting down to dinner. Before you begin, simply take a couple of minutes to make a note of what you appreciate about yourself.

I've noticed that some people have some resistance to this. You might not be used to thinking about yourself in this way, especially if you tend to concentrate on your limitations and weaknesses, rather than your strengths. If you feel hesitant, I encourage you to give it a go anyway. Try it for a week and then see how you feel. If it truly does nothing for you, ditch it. But if you think there might be some value to it, stick with it. Eventually it might become your favourite part of your day.

Show your appreciation for others

Are there people (or pets, as in my example above) who show up on your appreciation list? I bet there are.

Take a moment and tell those people that you appreciate them. Text them, phone them, do something to show them that you care.

Do me a favour and do this right now. Think of a person you appreciate. Now, go tell them you appreciate them. If they're not around, text, call or send them a quick email. It's enough to say, 'Hey, I was thinking about you today and I just want you to know that I appreciate you. Thanks for being you.'

That's it – that's all you have to do.

This simple act has a host of benefits. First of all, it deepens your appreciation, reminding you that you have people in your life that you are grateful for. This can take you out of tunnel-vision and remind you of how much you already have.

Second, it makes the other person feel good, expanding the impact of your appreciation and deepening your relationship, which I'll talk more about in a moment.

Third, helping others naturally makes us feel good. There's a reason that acts of service and volunteerism are recommended as a mental health strategy by experts. Doing good for others naturally makes us feel good and bolsters our self-esteem.

Avoid comparison

When I was sixteen and I started working out, Ja Rule was my inspiration. In case you aren't familiar with him, Ja Rule is an American rapper who was popular in the 1990s and early 2000s. At the height of his stardom, he was lean yet jacked, with impressive traps, biceps, abs and hip flexors – all of which he showed off by going shirtless and wearing his visible boxers low on his hips. He wore his baggy trousers even lower – it was the nineties after all.

When I tell people that Ja Rule was my inspiration, they usually laugh. What could a white boy living in Northern Ireland possibly have in common with a heavily tattooed, African American rapper from New York City? Nothing. And that's my point. Comparison is ridiculous, especially when we get into wishing for another person's arms, and another person's abs. We aren't Mr. Potato Head. We can't swap body parts. (Thank goodness – that would be weird.)

Comparing yourself to a celebrity is especially silly because actors are paid millions to prepare to look a certain way. They have dedicated nutritionists, trainers, private chefs and assistants, not to mention hair and make-up artists, to help them look a particular way for shoots.

Fitness models aren't that different. Models' bodies are their business, which means they put an incredible amount of time into looking a certain way, for a certain day. They organise their efforts around looking their best for a photo shoot. Once again, hair and make-up, good lighting, photo filters and airbrushing all play a role.

Most fitness models don't look 'cover-ready' all the time, either. This certainly was, and is, the case for me. Recently, I shared a shirtless photo of myself to highlight my first session back after over a week off. After I shared the photo on social media, someone reached out and asked me, 'Is that how you look all the time?'

It was a great question and one I was happy to answer honestly: *No*. The photo was taken after I'd been fasting for twelve hours (for most of which I was asleep) and I had just worked out so my muscles were popping. I was also under good lighting. And let's not forget, I've been working at this for twenty years; none of it happened overnight. But these are not the kinds of things you can tell from a photo.

Of course, if you are inspired by someone else, great. Ja Rule inspired me; he gave me the motivation to start working out and building muscle, and for that I thank him. But there's a difference between the occasional dash of

How to break the comparison habit

Comparing yourself to others can be a hard habit to break. Here are a few simple tips to disrupt the pattern:

Take time off social media. Social media can be a hotbed of comparison. Take a break from your usual social channels, or at least unfollow/mute people who tend to trigger your insecurity or comparison.

Humanise your heroes. Remind yourself that everyone wipes their own butt. Funny but true.

Challenge the myth of perfection. Remember that no one is perfect. Everyone you're comparing yourself to is a human being, and when it comes to human beings, there's no such thing as perfect. As I've said, chances are you wouldn't actually want to swap lives with them – especially if you knew what secret battles they're fighting.

Shift the focus back to your own life. Why worry about what other people are doing when you have your own life to lead? Put your time and energy into making the most of this very moment rather than wishing you could swap with someone else.

inspiration and chronic comparison. You will always be second best to the person you're comparing yourself to. It's much better to focus on yourself and your journey, rather than worrying about what other people are up to.

Practice: **Cultivate meaningful relationships**

Just before I began writing this book, I flew all the way to Canada to spend a week with a friend I've had since childhood, Callum. Given that we're both married and have busy careers, that might seem like a frivolous thing to do. And visiting Canada in January might seem like a dubious choice.

But to me it was an easy decision. Because friendship matters. We all know how good it feels to be among people who 'get us', and how lonely it feels to be disconnected or separated from loved ones for whatever reason. This was never more obvious than during the COVID-19 pandemic.

I visited Callum because I knew it would be good for my mental health, and for his. Winter can be long and dreary. The prospect of seeing a good friend who lives far away gave us both something to look forward to. Being with each other, getting goofy, even doing mundane things like running errands together did us both a world of good.

Yet relationships, particularly friendships, can fall onto the backburner of life. It's easy to take them for granted if you don't deliberately prioritise them. Friendship in particular can become more challenging as you get older – if you don't actively work at it. It can be easy to get drawn inwards, to focus only on your immediate family and your work, and let friendships fall to the wayside. But that only makes life smaller.

Luckily, you don't have to get on an international flight every time you want to connect with your loved ones. Even if your community is far flung, you can still make a point of interacting with friends virtually. Something I've learned is that you may have to be the one who initiates things; that's okay. Do it anyway. Make the phone call. Send the text. Suggest a time to hang out.

Don't wait; do it today. Better still, do it right now. That's another thing I learned from Mark: don't take your relationships for granted. Don't wait to tell someone you love them. You might not have another chance.

Phone a friend

This is so simple it almost sounds ridiculous to write it down. But it works.

Think about a loved one – someone you care about and wish you saw more of. Now, pick up the phone and call them.

If you really hate using the phone, you can send a text. But I encourage you to use the phone, because there's a closeness that happens when you hear the other person's voice and natural responses such as laughter that you don't get over text. You can use FaceTime or a virtual meeting if you prefer – but don't put it off.

And, while you're at it, tell them you love them. As I mentioned earlier, I started this practice a couple of years ago with my closest friends. Every time you tell someone you love them, you deepen your mutual connection a little more. And you give your brain a nice little dose of oxytocin and serotonin – two important feel-good hormones. Most of all, assuming they say it back, you feel loved. And nothing is better for your mental health that that.

Share your struggles

A little while ago I ran a coaching programme, a portion of which was specifically designed to help people take charge of their mental health and make small improvements, like the ones I'm telling you about in this book.

Shortly after it finished, a client, Craig, wrote to me and told me the programme had changed his life.

What was the life-changing part? Was it one of the habits or practices I'd assigned? No, as it turned out. Craig said that what made a difference to him was the way that I opened up about my own challenges. I'd shared stories similar to the ones you've been reading about: I expressed my own struggles, spoke to the sense of foreboding and fear I often have to work against, and explained how I treat mental health as an active practice to prevent myself from falling into the dark places that my brain might otherwise go.

Craig told me that it was my candour, my willingness to share, that inspired him. He, too, wanted to live with openness. He wanted to be willing to be vulnerable with others and share more of himself. Six months later, he came

The prospect of helping others is one of the biggest driving forces in my life; it pushes me to continue to look after myself, both mentally and physically.

out to his parents. After years of being closeted, he finally told his parents that he's gay. By coming out, he gave himself the opportunity to live truly, and fully as himself.

When Craig shared this with me – I'll be honest – I teared up. It meant so much to me to know that I'd helped someone else take such a meaningful leap. It was a humbling experience: a reminder that when we are willing to be honest and share something of ourselves, we not only give ourselves a chance to connect with other people, we just might inspire them to do the same thing. It's like a ripple effect.

Get extra support when you need it

When my dog, Ollie, gets sick, he hides. His natural instinct is to conceal his weakness so he isn't ousted from 'the pack'. If you're struggling, you might feel inclined to do the same thing – to say you're fine when you're not, to stop doing the things you usually do, to hide under the duvet. If so, that's understandable. But hiding from others is the exact opposite of what we should do in these moments. I tell my clients, when things get hard, please run *to* me – not *away from* me. While I can't fix things, I might be able to help. And if I can't help, I can at least be by your side while you're going through whatever you need to go through. That's what a coach is for.

If you're struggling with your mental health, remember that this is why therapists, psychologists, counsellors and doctors exist. Think of it this way: if your car has an issue, you take it to the mechanic. If your heart has an issue you go to the cardiologist. Why do we treat our mental health any differently? If your mental health requires a tune-up, talk to a professional.

Here's an added thing to remember if you're hesitant to open up or ask for help. Many people, myself included, consider it a gift to be able to help others. I bet you feel the same way. If a friend comes to you with a problem, and you're able to provide a shoulder to cry on or a listening ear, it makes you feel good, right? You're glad to have contributed in some way. That's how your friends and family will feel when you ask for a bit of support. Similarly, helping professionals tend to take pride in their work. They're there to help – they've chosen that profession for a reason. Personally, helping others has brought a great deal of depth and satisfaction to my life. Coaching makes me grateful to be alive. The prospect of helping others is one of the biggest driving forces in my life; it pushes me to continue to look after myself, both mentally and physically.

Finally, please remember that you're not alone. I have been to various mental health professionals over the years. My first experience was when I was just ten years old, after my granddad died. My mum noticed that I was feeling pretty down and struggling a bit in school, so she proactively arranged for me to see a counsellor.

I've since taken a page out of my mum's book and sought mental health support at various points in my life. For example, when my social media first blew up, I felt very overwhelmed. Suddenly I was speaking to over 100,000 people at a time, and I didn't want to say or do the wrong thing, nor did I want the experience to go to my head. Chatting with a psychologist helped put my mind at ease, and I came away with some tools to help me keep the experience in perspective.

More recently, when I began taking a new, revolutionary medication for cystic fibrosis (triple combination therapy), my medical team assigned me a psychologist to help me navigate any potential effects on my mental health.

I hope this helps take the stigma out of seeking support. Remember, other people care about you and want you to be well. Don't hesitate to do what you need for your mental health, because you matter.

Summary

We all have limitations in our lives. Some of them are changeable, some are not. And that's okay. 'Fitness without limits' doesn't mean you never have any limitations on yourself whatsoever. It means you keep you moving forward anyway.

Mental health is an essential component of that approach. No, you won't be positive and happy all the time – no one is. But if you care for your mental health regularly, you will find that you're better able to handle whatever comes, that you keep making progress despite obstacles, and that you can actually enjoy and appreciate the process (at least some of the time).

Many of the limitations and losses you'll experience in this life are beyond your control. But you can always choose to actively care for your mental health. That's a choice worth making, again and again.

And when in doubt, just breathe.

 RECAP

Your key mental health practices are:

- Breathe
- Foster appreciation
- Cultivate meaningful relationships

PRINCIPLE #4: MOVEMENT

When I was about twelve, I thought I would be clever and use my CF to my advantage. If I didn't feel like participating in PE, I'd tell the teacher that I was having trouble breathing or that my stomach hurt and, since the faculty was aware of my condition, the teacher would immediately grant me a pass and I could sit out.

After trying this a few times, however, I realised that I wasn't actually benefitting from sitting out. I wound up feeling bored and alone. More than that, even though I'd faked the excuse, sitting out made me feel somehow less capable than my peers, as if the lie had become real. After trying this a few times (usually when the weather was particularly bad), it became clear to me that by avoiding physical education I wasn't getting away with something, I was only doing myself a disservice.

Luckily, I clued in. My mindset shifted there and then. I decided it was better to work with and around my condition – to do as much as I possibly could – than use it as a reason to avoid things. Since then, I've never used my CF as an excuse to miss out on life. If anything, I use it as a reason to make sure I'm in the game, not on the sidelines. And that means moving my body as much as I can, any way I can.

These days, I'm a huge advocate for movement of all kinds. Human beings are designed to move. If we sit around too much, our bodies start to suffer – but give us an opportunity to move and we thrive. A sedentary human is like a bird in a cage. When we prevent ourselves from moving regularly, we're only caging ourselves. Movement, on the other hand, sets us free.

To become better at moving in general, we first need to uncouple 'exercise' from 'movement'. Exercise involves movement, but movement doesn't have to involve exercise. Exercise is something you do intentionally. When you exercise, you go to the gym and lift weights or take a group fitness class. Exercise is important, but it actually represents a very small piece of the puzzle in regard to physical fitness. Think about it: if you exercise for an hour, that is 4 per cent of your day. Just 4 per cent! Sure, it's a valuable 4 per cent, but what's more important is how you spend the remaining 96 per cent.

That's where movement comes in. Movement refers to however else you move your body. Movement is what happens when you cook a meal, walk the dog, vacuum your apartment, run to catch a bus, or struggle to put pants on your toddler. Movement is kicking a ball around the garden with your kid, carrying your groceries home from the shops, or dancing around with all the confidence of a child in a Superman T-shirt. This kind of movement might not seem like much, but it matters. And the more you can do, the better.

How much movement you get in through the course of the day will of course depend on how you spend your time. Some people have active jobs where they are already moving around a lot. If you're a nurse, you're likely on your feet all day as you move around the hospital and attend to patients. If you're a dog walker or a mail carrier, you're walking for a good portion of the day. If you're a manual labourer or tradesperson, you're likely very active on a regular basis. On the other hand, many folks have desk jobs where their work involves quite a bit of sitting down. Chances are, if you're reading this book, you're looking for ways to move more – and if so, it's useful to consider something called NEAT.

Movement is NEAT

NEAT – or Non-Exercise Activity Thermogenesis – refers to energy expenditure that takes place outside of structured exercise. It's the energy (i.e. calories) you burn through movement that happens naturally throughout the course of the day. This can include activity such as walking, doing housework, doing whatever your job involves – say, moving around the classroom if you're a teacher, or making coffee if you're a barista – or even movement you don't notice such as fidgeting or gesturing.

While these calories might not seem like much, they can really add up. The more active you are throughout the course of your day, the more calories you'll burn from NEAT. For example, NEAT can account for 15–30 per cent of your daily calorie expenditure.

Clearly, increasing your NEAT throughout the day can make a big difference to your overall fitness level, and it can improve your results – especially if your goal is to create a calorie deficit and encourage fat loss. Think of it not as a replacement for exercise, but a powerful upgrade.

To gain an idea of where your current activity lies, here are some ballpark figures to keep in mind:

- ▶ Under 5,000 steps per day = Low activity
- ▶ 5,000-7,500 steps per day = Moderate activity
- ▶ 7,500-10,000 steps per day = High activity
- ▶ 10,000+ steps = Very high activity

In a moment, I'll share some practices that will help you move more and get more NEAT in your life. But first, I want to acknowledge that for many people, being told to simply 'move more' isn't enough. First, we have to address some common roadblocks that might be preventing you from getting more movement in your life. Let's tackle them one by one.

Common roadblock #1: 'I have a physical limitation'

A friend of mine recently offered me a fancy SLR camera that he no longer wanted. He knew that I've been using a less versatile compact camera to create my Warhammer YouTube videos and assumed I'd jump at the chance to upgrade.

To his surprise, I declined. I explained to him that I know exactly how my current camera works, and exactly how to make it do what I want it to do. It's not the best camera out there, but I've figured out how to make the most of it, so it works for me.

Bodies are similar. You may have physical limitations – injuries, illnesses, conditions or particular needs that require special care or consideration. That's how human bodies are; 'perfect' doesn't exist. It doesn't make sense to wish away our physical limitations or unique requirements. What's far better is to work with our bodies, understand them, and adapt accordingly.

This reminds me of my client Gianna, whose arms had been amputated at the elbow. She refused to let this stand in her way. Instead, she adapted her workouts and made the most of what she could do. We concluded our coaching after she made the decision to start training for the Paralympics in the cycling category.

It's not about the limitation, but what you do with it. The person who embraces and works with their physical limitations will be able to do far more than a person who has no physical limitations but who doesn't know themselves and isn't willing to do the work necessary to grow. Progress, in other words, isn't about having the perfect body or zero obstacles. Progress belongs to the person who is willing to work with what they have.

More reasons to move

Remember how I told you that sleep is like a wonder drug? Well, movement is another one.

Regular movement is linked to both longevity and quality of life. It's known to support overall physical function and wellness including heart health, brain function and brain health, bone density, digestive function, energy levels, mental health and more. At the same time, it can also reduce risk of concerns such as cardiovascular disease, type 2 diabetes, strokes, cancer . . . need I go on?

It boils down to this: anything you want your body to do, movement will help your body do it better. And that includes all the other principles you read about in this book. Physical activity has been shown to contribute to better sleep, better digestion and better mental health. So if you're trying to work on any of the things we've discussed so far – sleep, nutrition or mental health – movement will only make your efforts easier and more effective.

If you have a limitation of some kind, I encourage you to avoid focusing on what's *not* possible, and divert all your attention and effort to what *is* possible. What can you do? What might you be able to do with some additional support, modifications, or creativity? What kinds of workarounds can you come up with? Who could you ask for help to make it happen?

Remember: you are a problem solver. You have what it takes to figure out solutions and options for yourself. Don't take yourself out of the game – find a way in.

Common roadblock #2: 'But I'm not a fitness person!'

As you read this book, you might have a slight concern at the back of your mind that fitness – including movement – just isn't for you.

Maybe you're thinking, 'But I'm not a fitness person!' If you've never been particularly active, or you've been overweight your entire life, the idea of becoming physically active might feel foreign or even at odds with your identity, your sense of who you are.

If so, I can relate. And not just because I didn't think of myself as a 'fitness person' growing up. If you were to meet me now, you'd likely peg me as an extraverted, outgoing kind of guy. A 'people person'. And you'd be right: I make friends with people pretty easily, I try to be personable with people I encounter, and I usually feel relaxed in most social situations.

But when I was younger, I was completely different. Throughout my entire childhood right through to my time in secondary school, I was extremely shy. If I got called upon in class, I would turn beetroot red, my eyes would start watering and I'd start sweating profusely. I wore layers of shirts each day knowing I would sweat right through them. I could barely speak to people other than my friends and family. As you can imagine, I was uncomfortable and nervous quite a lot of the time.

When I left secondary school and enrolled on the National Diploma programme at sixteen, I walked into a brand-new environment. No one in the programme knew me – everyone was a stranger. This could have made me extremely anxious and triggered all my usual shy behaviours. But on the first day of class I had a realisation: no one here knew me.

> ## You'll be amazed at the progress you make when you simply decide to be the person you want to be.

They didn't know I was shy. They didn't know I was awkward. They didn't even know I had CF. For all they knew, I was a sporty, cool, confident guy.

I saw an opportunity to re-invent myself, and I took it.

I decided to be the guy I wanted to be. I took all my old stories about who I was and who I couldn't be and pushed them to the side. I struck up conversations and joked and laughed. I put my hand up in class. I started working out and got more involved in rugby.

Amazingly, the sweating, eye-watering and blushing stopped. The 'fake it till you make it' approach worked. The more I talked to people, the more comfortable I became in social situations. Before I knew it, I was no longer 'faking it'. I simply outgrew my shyness and genuinely became a social person who was relatively comfortable in his own skin. To be clear, it wasn't that I was pretending to be someone I wasn't or trying to fit in. I simply gave myself the chance for a fresh start: to show up the way I wanted to show up.

Sometimes, we get locked into an old identity without realising it. We fall into ways of doing things and believe certain things about who we are and who we have to be, simply because that's the way we've always done them, or that's the way we've always been. But your past doesn't have to dictate your future.

A really amazing thing about identity and our sense of self is that it's changeable. At any point on any given day, you can decide who to be. You can choose to change a part of who you are. That doesn't mean change is easy; it can be challenging to break habits, learn new skills and practise unfamiliar things. But the decision is always possible. And once you've made the decision, you've opened up the door to something new.

If you don't think of yourself as a fit person, consider revising that script right now. Suppose you decided this very second that you *are* a fit person. What might you do differently? What choices might you make today? How would 'fit person you' find more ways to move throughout the course of their day?

You'll be amazed at the progress you make when you simply decide to be the person you want to be.

Common roadblock #3: 'I'm afraid to get out of my comfort zone'

I promise that you have possibilities within yourself that you have not yet discovered. I want you to discover those possibilities: to discover just how much you're capable of, just how resilient you are, just how much potential you possess.

The cliché that life happens at the end of your comfort zone is true. Some of the most memorable, beautiful experiences of your life will occur outside of your comfort zone. It really is where the best stuff happens.

If you only stay where you feel comfortable and safe, you're limiting yourself. You're preventing yourself from experiencing the fullness of what you can do. On the other hand, when you believe in yourself, when you are willing to take yourself out of your comfort zone, that's where you become truly limitless.

Having said that, 'get out of your comfort zone' isn't the most helpful advice. The truth is, people rarely blast through their comfort zones all at once. Rather, testing your limits in small doses and slowly nudging yourself out of your comfort zone tends to work better. When you increase your confidence over time, your willingness to try difficult things and your physical capability and tolerance for difficult things will increase.

To do that, here's a strategy I like to use.

First, whenever you begin something, such as a new exercise routine or a new activity, judge how comfortable you feel with it on a scale of 0 to 10. From there, get in some practice with whatever the new activity or routine is. As you go, periodically check in with yourself regarding your comfort level. With more time and practice, you'll probably notice your comfort level increases. Once your comfort level reaches 5/10 or higher, it's probably time to increase your discomfort level. You might do that by increasing the intensity, frequency or duration of a task – or try something new altogether.

Here's an example. Let's say you want to start walking more. Perhaps it's not particularly comfortable for you: you feel out of breath, your knees hurt and you feel conspicuous walking down the street. On the plus side, you do know how to walk, and you own a pair of trainers, so you're not completely uncomfortable. Let's say you gauge your comfort level as 1/10.

Now assume you start walking on a regular basis, and after a few weeks of taking daily walks, you start to feel a bit more comfortable. Let's say your knees still hurt but you feel a little less breathless and a bit more familiar with your route, so you'd rank your comfort level at 3/10.

Over time, with continued walking, you start to see your comfort level grow. Perhaps by a couple of months of consistent walking you rank your comfort level at 6/10. You know your route, your knees hurt less, you don't feel as breathless, and you're too busy enjoying listening to your podcast or playlist to worry about what other people might be thinking. Great: now you can increase the discomfort level a bit.

To amp up the discomfort, you might walk a little longer, a little faster and/ or add a new route. You might even want to sign up for a 5k charity walk, or try something new altogether, like running or cycling. Congratulations, you've now expanded your comfort zone!

The point here is to continue to challenge yourself as your comfort grows. As you can see, you don't have to jump right into the deep end of the pool and do the scariest thing you can think of. But you will want to continually nudge yourself out of your comfort zone so you don't get stuck.

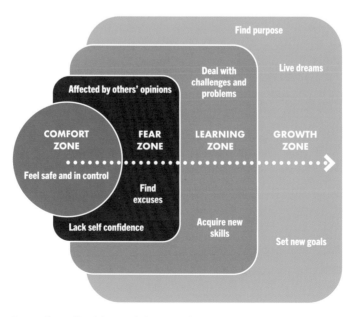

Source: https://positivepsychology.com/comfort-zone/

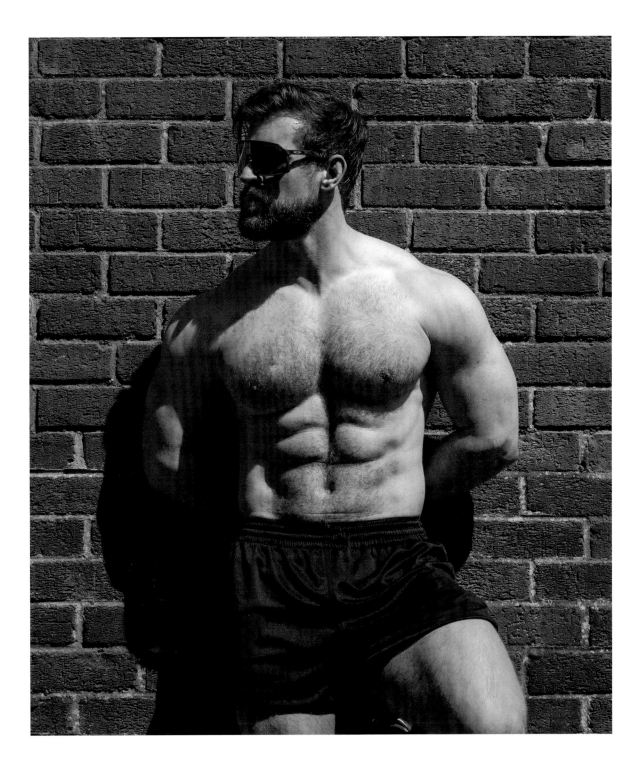

An additional caveat here: as you approach new things, remember that you likely won't be good at things that are brand new to you. You may indeed look very silly. I probably looked completely ridiculous the first few times I tried slacklining; I fell off more times than I could count. (For that matter, I was quite a sight hanging upside down from the harness while highlining. And that's just what you could see. I promise you I had the biggest wedgie imaginable while clinging to those ropes for dear life.)

Your mindset is powerful. Choose to focus on the effort you're putting in rather than the results. I like to tell myself that getting to the starting line is a win in itself.

The more you rack up small wins, the more you'll be able to build new skills and cultivate new abilities, and the more you'll be able to tackle new things with confidence. So, start small and work on developing your abilities a bit each time. As small wins stack up, you'll be able to strive for bigger, more daunting goals.

Movement practices

With all that in mind, how can you incorporate more movement into your daily life so you can build up your base of fitness, burn more energy and increase your confidence?

I'm so glad you asked. My key practices for movement are as follows:

- Increase your step count
- Look for the adventure
- Embrace an 'always something' approach

Practice: Increase your step count

Step count is a useful metric as a gauge of your overall movement. By tracking your daily steps, you can get a general idea of how active or sedentary you are. People tend to focus on exact numbers – such as getting in 10,000 steps – but the truth is, exact numbers don't matter so much. What matters is your own personal progress. Increasing your steps on average is more important than achieving some arbitrary number.

I like focusing on steps because, while walking is by no means the only form of movement, it is a pretty good one. Walking offers loads of health benefits, including supporting cardiovascular fitness, lowering blood pressure, improving circulation, reducing risk of chronic disease, contributing to good mental health and more.

Here are some ways you can increase your daily steps.

Track your steps

You can track your steps using a pedometer, a smart watch or an app on your phone. As with calories, it's the average that matters most here rather than any single day. I recommend tracking your steps over the course of a week. Tally up your daily step count, divide it by seven, and you'll have a weekly average.

Once you have your weekly average, aim to increase that number just a little bit the following week. Continue to increase your steps week by week, or at least maintain your steps if that's more reasonable, depending on how much you're moving.

Don't worry too much about the accuracy of a given step-counter. As I said, it's not the number that matters, it's the progress. Even if your step-counter is inaccurate, if you're consistent with it, you'll still get a pretty good picture of your progress. The trick is to choose one step-counter and stick with it. If you use a Garmin one day and your phone's 'Health' app the next, then you might not have a reliable picture of your steps because each counter will measure things slightly differently. But if you pick one and use it consistently, you'll know whether your steps are increasing or decreasing, and that's the measurement that matters.

Look for sneaky ways to add in more steps

If you're able to add a long walk to each day that's great – but it isn't essential. In fact, most people will benefit more from sneaking in steps throughout the day. When you get into the mindset of 'a few more steps', you'll start to discover how quickly they can add up.

Here's an example. Suppose you're at the gym waiting for a machine. You could just stand there and wait. Or you could pace around while you're

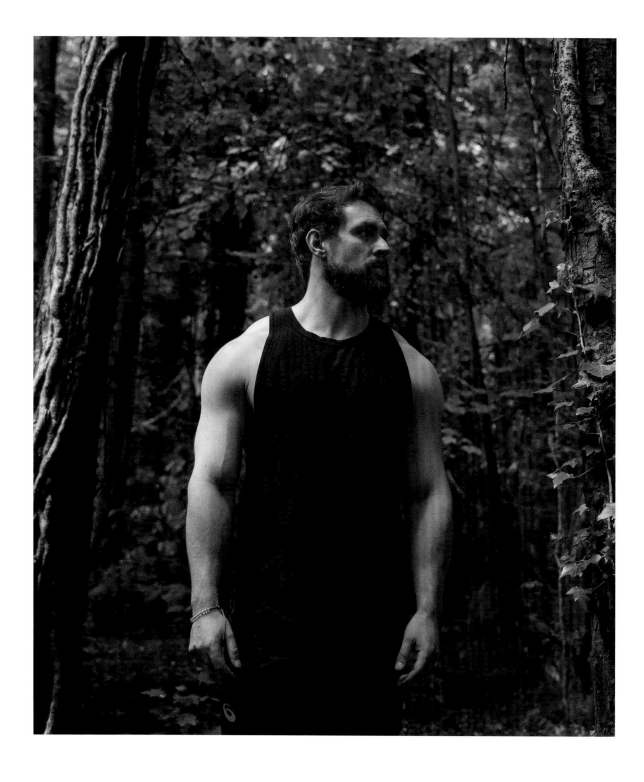

waiting. Let's say you get in an extra thirty steps that way. Admittedly, thirty steps is not a lot. But suppose you do that every time you wait for a machine, which might be five times per workout. That's 150 steps. If you exercise three times a week, that's 450 steps. Over the course of a year, that's 25,200 extra steps you wouldn't otherwise have taken. That's roughly how many steps you'd take to walk a half marathon!

Practice: **Look for the adventure**

Fitness is often about doing the mundane so that you can do the extraordinary. Physical fitness is like possessing a key: it can unlock doors. It's a gateway to doing some pretty cool stuff. But on a daily basis, it often means doing things that are kinda boring. And while there's nothing wrong with that, it can help to bring in a bit of adventurousness to your regular movement. Here are a couple of options to try.

Take a new path

Humans are creatures of habit. We tend to walk the same routes, day after day. But getting off the beaten track – literally and figuratively – can make daily movement more enticing and rewarding.

Just recently I went for a hike with my wife, sister-in-law, mother-in-law and our dogs. We were all set to take the usual route when I paused and said, 'Hey, how about we take the path through the forest instead?'

Everyone agreed and we set off on our mini-adventure. The forest was a new landscape to us, and a bit more challenging as the terrain was more hilly and less travelled. We worked up a bit of a sweat climbing over fallen logs and manoeuvring around the bushes and branches. The dogs loved it too. The entire experience was more fun and engaging – for our bodies and our minds – than simply walking on autopilot around the usual route.

Next time you go for a walk, look for a slightly different route. If you walk in a town or city, try walking along roads you've not been down before, or go one block further than you usually go. If you typically take the bus, try getting off one stop later than normal. If you enjoy nature walks, pick a path that's less familiar to you.

Of course, this doesn't just apply to walking. Your 'new path' might mean trying yoga or tennis for the first time. It might mean checking out a dance class. It might mean hopping on your bicycle and exploring an unfamiliar neighbourhood. And remember, small movements matter too: perhaps you want to try knitting or painting to give your hands something to do while you watch television. Or you could try cooking a new recipe or walking to a new restaurant instead of grabbing your standard takeaway. The important thing is to mix things up. The more new stuff you try, the more movement you're likely to include in your day – and the more fun you'll have along the way.

Add a soundtrack

Music can add a new dimension to otherwise monotonous situations. Make yourself a playlist of songs to get you moving, such as a 'midday dance break' or 'errand-running tunes'. If you really want to get nerdy with this, here's a fun trick to turn your regular walks into bold quests: add an epic soundtrack. Go for a walk or hike to *The Lord of the Rings* score, and I promise your ramble will feel like a grand adventure.

Practice: Embrace an 'always something' approach

Sometimes clients tell me they are perfectionists. When I hear that word, my immediate reaction is 'uh oh'.

Perfectionism – or an 'all or nothing' mentality – puts a wall between you and progress. It puts a whole bunch of limits on what you can do. Life isn't perfect, bodies aren't perfect, people aren't perfect . . . the whole idea of perfectionism is a myth.

If you're stuck on perfect, I have, er, the 'perfect' antidote for you. Instead of aiming for the optimal, ideal way of doing things, focus instead on an 'always something' approach.

Here's an example. When I was stuck in the hospital with a line in my arm, I looked for teeny tiny bits of movement I could do. My one arm was largely incapacitated but there was nothing stopping me from working out my other arm. I looked around my room and noticed the metal bin, so I grabbed that and did some single-arm lateral raises a couple of times a day. That might sound silly – had a nurse peered into my room while I was lifting the bin

I'm sure they would have thought, *What on earth is this guy doing?* – but I knew that sneaking in some movement would give me a small sense of accomplishment when I felt otherwise disempowered and bored. Plus, I knew that some small and relatively gentle movement would facilitate my recovery and help me get back to normal once I finally left the hospital.

I've learned through my own experiences and from those around me that there's nearly always something you can do. And when you take an 'always something' approach, you can't *not* make progress. Here are some ways to put that 'always something' attitude into action.

Make an oath or personal pact

A while ago back, I took a personal oath to always take the stairs, unless I absolutely cannot do it. This has made for some interesting moments, such as traversing some immensely long flights of stairs on the London Underground while juggling heavy luggage. But this oath has served me well as I'm able to climb stairs quite quickly and comfortably, and I know it contributes to my overall fitness. Plus, it's satisfying; I take a little bit of pride in knowing I take the slightly more challenging route whenever it's available.

Consider making a personal pact of your own that suits your interests and activity level. For example, if you take the bus to and from work each day, you might commit to getting off one stop before your destination. If you typically take the lift at work, you could commit to taking the stairs – if not all the time, then on certain days or times of the week. Or you could commit to taking a short walk each day, even if it's just for three minutes, no matter the weather.

You might be surprised at how satisfying it can feel to do something a little outside of the norm. While most people are packing into a crowded lift or bus, you'll be proud of yourself for putting in the extra effort and going your own way.

Look for 'small bites'

When you bite off more than you can chew, you inevitably have to spit out what you've bitten off, leaving you with nothing. It's much better to take small bites. Not just when it comes to food, though that's a pretty good idea too, but when it comes to tackling movement goals.

As an alternative to big bites (i.e. big, daunting movement goals you're unlikely to achieve), seek out 'movement nibbles' – manageable little bits of movement you can snack on throughout the day. For example, do a few air squats while you wait for your coffee to brew. Pace around while you're on a phone call. Walk to the corner shop rather than driving. Put on your favourite song and jump around for a while. Or, like me, take the stairs rather than the escalator or lift.

Small bites might seem like nothing in the moment, but don't underestimate them. Little efforts, the kind that are so simple and easy you barely notice them, stack up. When you put them all together, they can have a significant impact on your body, your health, and your results. Keep watch throughout your day for possible movement nibbles, and snack on them as often as you like.

Pick lower-hanging fruit

A while ago, I took up swimming. Friends of mine who also swim had loads of advice on the best pools to go to and the optimal times to swim. The difference between their 'optimal' approach and my reality was laughable. I swam at a busy leisure centre. The pool was designed for families, not for serious training. The lanes were narrow and the pool was mostly filled with kids, laughing and splashing about. The water wasn't deep; at the shallow end of the pool my knees practically hit the floor as I swam.

Did I quit going and find a better pool like my friends suggested? Absolutely not. Because the leisure centre was on my way home from work. It wasn't the best pool in the world, but it was accessible and allowed me to sneak in a quick swim without hugely changing my daily routine. If I had to drive across the city to some other pool, I wouldn't have time and I'd have to quit swimming altogether. The convenience factor was essential.

That's what I mean by picking lower-hanging fruit. Look for stuff that is doable, accessible and relatively easy. The easier you make it on yourself, the more likely it is to happen.

Think about what you have access to and consider how you might make the most of it. Sure, you might prefer to go for a gorgeous hill walk on a Sunday afternoon, but during the week maybe a stroll around your neighbourhood will suffice. Perhaps you'd love to plan a visit to the botanical gardens, but in

Could you lose 30 lbs in just three minutes a day?

One day I got a message from Aaron, a client who'd been working with me for a couple of months.

According to his text message, Aaron was feeling defeated and wanted to quit.

When I hopped onto a video call with him, he sighed. 'I'm sorry, Ben,' he said. 'I just haven't got the time to go to the gym and do all this stuff. Between work and life stuff, it's hard to keep up and I'm feeling rather bad about myself.'

I said to him, 'Okay, Aaron. How about this. Can you walk for three minutes?'

Aaron looked at me like I was nuts. 'What?' he said.

'Can you walk for three minutes? Even just around your house.'

'Of course I can,' he said.

'Okay, then. Once a day, I want you to put on your favourite song, walk around for three minutes, then have a glass of water. Text me a photo of the empty glass. Can you do that?'

'Sure,' he repeated. 'No problem. What else should I do?'

'That's it,' I said. 'Just do that. Trust me. Do that for a week, and then we'll check in again.'

Aaron followed the plan to the letter. One week later, we agreed that he'd continue with the daily three-minute plan for the following week, but this time on one of those days he would walk for five minutes rather than three.

Over time, we increased Aaron's walks – he began walking for fifteen minutes, then twenty minutes, and so on.

Six months later, Aaron had lost 14 kilos (30 lbs) and he told me he felt 'energetic and amazing'.

Did just a few minutes of daily walking transform his body? Of course not. With time, he also employed the other practices you've been learning about in this book, including adjusting his calorie intake and hitting the gym when he was able. But the approach of small, daily effort eliminated the overwhelm and gave him a sense of achievement that allowed him to build a solid foundation. If we hadn't kept things simple, Aaron would have stopped altogether. By emphasising small efforts, he was able to keep going – and that's what matters the most.

Little efforts, no matter how small, add up to big results.

the meantime, you can tend to a little garden patch at home. Can't get to yoga class on busy weeknights? Do a few stretches at home, or try a virtual class. You get the idea. Life is complicated enough; keep things simple by doing what you can, when you can.

Summary

Exercise is great; no denying that. In fact, in the next part of the book, I'll walk you through my programming principles so you can make the most of your workouts.

But as you've now learned, exercise is just one very small piece of the puzzle. Your overall activity level matters – and by simply increasing your daily movement, you can radically improve your fitness, your health, your energy levels and your results, such as losing body fat if you so desire.

Don't get stuck in thinking your movement has to be 'all or nothing'. Find small, simple ways to move throughout your day and increase your step count. Remember: you're a problem solver. Be creative, and have fun coming up with clever ways to sneak movement into your day.

For many people, movement can feel uncomfortable at first. You might feel like you're not a fit person or that physical activity isn't for you. I promise you: movement is your birthright. The human body is designed to move, and no matter your starting point, you can move more and move better over time, if you keep at it.

Whatever limitations or obstacles you face, I have confidence that you can find workarounds and solutions to make movement possible and doable for yourself. Work with things as they are, rather than waiting for them to be perfect. Nudge yourself further and further from your comfort zone. Before you know it, your current comfort zone will feel like a tiny dot in the distance You'll have endless possibilities at your fingertips, and you'll know that your potential is truly limitless.

↻ RECAP

Your key movement practices are:

- Increase your step count
- Look for the adventure
- Embrace an 'always something' approach

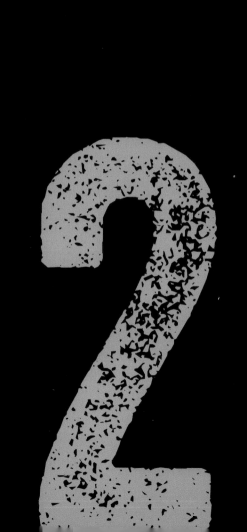

PART TWO

EXERCISE PROGRAMMING

At sixteen years old, when I first started working out with our home 'multigym' machine, I had no idea what I was doing. The machine came with a long list of potential exercises you could do on it – probably thirty in total. I'd go out to our garage, put on some music (usually Ja Rule), and go through the list, doing each exercise one-by-one until I'd completed all of them.

Everyone is a beginner at some point

After a few months of using the multigym, my friend Callum and I decided to go the gym and try working out 'for real'. While I'd started to build up some muscle and strength from my at-home workouts, the actual gym felt intimidating to me. That's the real reason Callum and I went together: we were both too chicken to go on our own.

Walking onto the gym floor, we both stopped and stared. Where to begin? There were so many strange machines and gadgets. I pointed to one crazy-looking contraption and muttered to Callum, 'What the heck does that do?'

Over the course of multiple visits (and enlisting some members of the staff to help us) we started to figure things out. Of course, being silly teenagers, Callum and I only cared about the body parts you could see in the mirror. We completely ignored important muscle groups like our back muscles and glutes in favour of repeatedly working our arms, chest and abs.

In time, of course, my knowledge and skills developed, and I eventually started learning about human physiology and exercise science. The better I trained, the more my body responded. When you're a newcomer to fitness, or if you haven't exercised in a long time, your body is like a sponge – it responds remarkably well to the new stimulus. I probably put on about 14 kilos (30 lbs) of muscle in that first year. While that is unusually high, it does demonstrate the immense potential you have when just starting out. The phenomenon is sometimes called 'beginner magic', referring to the fact that a person's

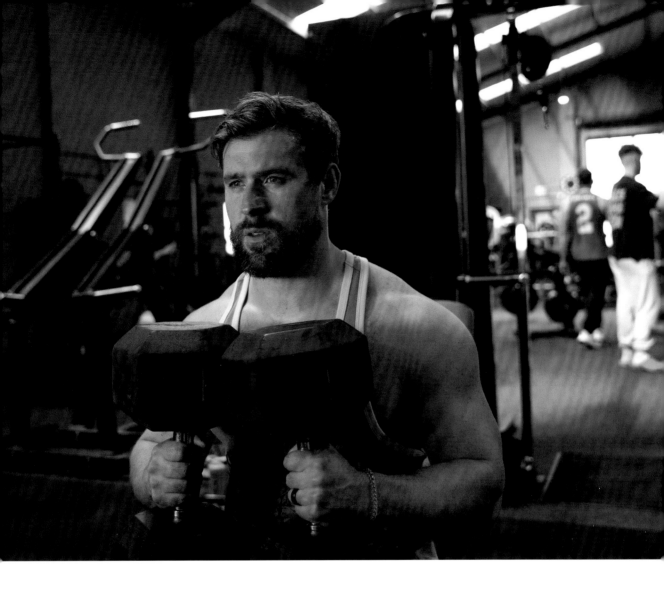

greatest gains or improvements tend to happen within their first six months to a year of exercising.

If you feel in any way uncertain, overwhelmed or doubtful about exercising in the gym, I hope my story reassures you somewhat. I know what it's like to have zero confidence in your body. But I also know what it's like to discover that your body can do more than you imagined, to realise that you are stronger than you think, and that you are more capable than you thought. I also know what it's like to see your body change. Seeing my quads, biceps and chest muscles develop was amazing to me. Appreciating the physical appearance of your body isn't necessarily vain. In my case, it served as a visual representation of breaking through my own limitations. I wasn't just gaining muscle; I was building a suit of armour. I was protecting myself from cystic fibrosis, and in the process, re-envisioning myself as someone far more powerful than I'd ever imagined myself to be.

This is why I am so passionate about what I do, and why I would encourage you to give resistance training a try, even if you're hesitant: because I know how revolutionary it can be. If you show up and put the work in, you'll be amazed at what can happen. In time, your confidence will build, your self-perception will evolve, and you'll open endless doors for yourself.

If resistance training or lifting weights has felt off-limits to you, let me assure you, it isn't. You don't have to have a fancy, expensive gym membership – your basic neighbourhood gym should have everything you need. You don't need to dedicate tons of time to train; you can work with whatever you've got, even if that means starting with just one session a week. And you don't have to follow complicated, convoluted programmes or methods. The system I'm about to lay out is highly adaptable and flexible to any situation, and you can scale things up or down depending on your preferences, abilities and comfort level.

Here's a look at what we'll cover in this section of the book:

Section A: Resistance training 101

Here I'll address why resistance training matters, and I'll outline five core principles to guide your training. I'll also bust a few myths, showing you why resistance training can be easier and more attainable than you might think.

Section B: Structuring your workouts

In this section I'll introduce you to compound movements, outline three types of workouts, and provide a fun method to make your workouts quicker and more effective.

Section C: Scheduling and supporting your programme

Next, I'll help you determine how often you should exercise, how to make the most of your time at the gym, and how to incorporate recovery and other activities into your life.

Let's dive in.

SECTION A: RESISTANCE TRAINING 101

Why resistance training matters

Resistance training, which is sometimes called weight training or strength training, is just as it sounds: you train the body by demanding your muscles work against a competing force or weight – i.e. resistance. This can involve machines, dumbbells, barbells or even bodyweight movements.

Previously, I explained that exercise doesn't have to take over your whole life. As I've said, if you exercise for one hour, that represents only 4 per cent of your day. And that's assuming you spend an entire hour exercising, which, as you'll see, isn't always necessary. Nonetheless, while exercise represents a small part of your day, it's also a very important part. Think of it like bicarbonate of soda (or baking powder) in a cake. You typically only need a tiny amount, but if you forget to include it, your cake won't rise. It's a small but imperative ingredient.

Resistance training is valuable for a host of reasons. As I discussed in Part One, it's beneficial purely as a form of movement. The sheer act of getting yourself moving around and getting your heart rate up will do you good. But there's more to it than that. Importantly, it helps you build strength and physical capability. Lift weights regularly, and you'll discover that things that felt more difficult before – like picking up your kids, carrying your luggage or even squatting down to tie your shoes – now feel easier and more natural.

If you want to make changes to your body composition, such as reducing body fat and/or gaining muscle, resistance training will play a significant role in helping you do so. Want to build muscle? Lifting weights, when paired with adequate recovery (i.e. nutrition and sleep) is arguably essential. Want fat loss? Resistance training can contribute by slightly increasing your metabolic rate over time.

But wait, there's more! Resistance training offers a host of health benefits. To name a few, it decreases the risk of chronic disease; supports brain, bone and heart health; decreases the risk of falls and injury; and supports better physical functioning, longevity and quality of life. It's a smart thing to do for your health, especially as you age – and the best time to start is now.

Having said all that, I think the single most important reason to strength train is that it gives you a deep-down feeling of confidence. Lifting weights is a force multiplier in this sense. The stronger you get, the more confidence you have in yourself, your body and your abilities. And the more confidence you have, the more you're able and willing to take on greater challenges, get out of your comfort zone and expand your horizons. Your perceived limitations will dissolve before your eyes.

Recently, my wife and I took a trip to Spain. While there, we decided to check out a nearby gym. When we walked in, we had every reason to be intimidated: it was packed full of people, they had loads of high-end equipment, and it was an unfamiliar space in a country where we don't speak the language. Yet I felt at home. I've now spent enough time in fitness environments that they feel natural to me. More importantly, I feel completely confident in my abilities. This gives me a sense of ease that I would have given anything for when I was younger. And that kind of confidence is possible for you, too.

Exercise is for everyone. You deserve to move your body and experience all the good things that come from that. As with everything else you've learned in this book, resistance training does not require perfection. You don't have to change who you are or completely overhaul your lifestyle to do it. You can show up to the gym exactly as you are and give it your best shot. You can adapt your exercise programming into a system and schedule that works for you and your lifestyle. Keep reading and I'll show you how to exercise, how to get the best return on your investment of time and energy, and ultimately, how make it work for *you*.

Five principles of resistance training

When it comes right down to it, effective resistance training depends on five key principles. Focus on this handful of things and you'll be able to exercise effectively and efficiently with minimal stress, complication or confusion.

While all of these principles matter, some are more important than others. As with your nutrition practices, you can imagine these as a pyramid. Focus primarily on the foundational principles within the pyramid, and you'll have a strong base. From there, you can drill down into some of the finer details.

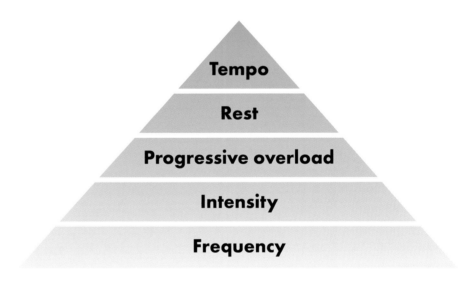

Principle #1: **Frequency**

When it comes to frequency, there are two considerations.

The first thing you have to do is show up. That sounds funny, but it's true. Often, the hardest part of going to the gym is just going to the gym. I'll talk more about scheduling in a moment; as you'll learn, you don't have to exercise every single day, and more is not necessarily better. Nonetheless, getting to the gym with some degree of consistency or regular frequency is vital to make progress. Whether that's once a week or four times a week, simply showing up and coming back is where the magic happens.

The second thing to consider is frequency of movement. When you start doing certain exercises, you need to stick to them for a while. Doing the same exercises on a regular basis will help you gain proficiency, minimise stress, reduce cognitive effort and help you avoid the awkward dance of pretending you know what you're doing while trying to remember how exactly that machine works. The more familiar you are with your exercise routine, the better you can focus on the physical task at hand.

In practical terms, this means sticking to a programme for about six weeks at a time, rather than doing something different every time you walk into the gym. If you've been doing the same workout for six weeks and you're ready for a change (maybe you're getting bored, there's always a queue for the machine you want to use, or you've reached a plateau where you aren't making many improvements), then you can make an adjustment. But ideally, you'll change as little as possible. Feel free to mix up a movement here or there, but if an exercise is working for you, don't change it.

(As a bonus, consistent frequency with both gym attendance and repeated exercises will also help with Principle #3: Progressive overload.)

Principle #2: Intensity

If it doesn't challenge you, it doesn't change you. This is the principle of intensity in a nutshell.

As much as getting to the gym is the first step, it's also possible to spend time in the gym without really *doing* anything. To make the most of your time there, you need to push yourself. Effort (aka intensity) is what creates change.

Effort is between you and you. I'm not here to judge whether you're giving 'enough' effort. That's something you need to decide for yourself. Further, effort will change from day to day. If you're stressed out, overtired and feeling down one day, your best effort might look like a walk on the treadmill. If you're feeling okay but a little 'meh', it might mean going through the motions of your routine with lighter weights; maybe once you get moving you'll discover you have more effort to give than you thought. On the other hand, if you're feeling energetic and up for a challenge, you can take that opportunity to add on some extra weight, and maybe even chase a personal best. It all depends on the situation. The important thing is to give your best effort each day, whatever that looks like.

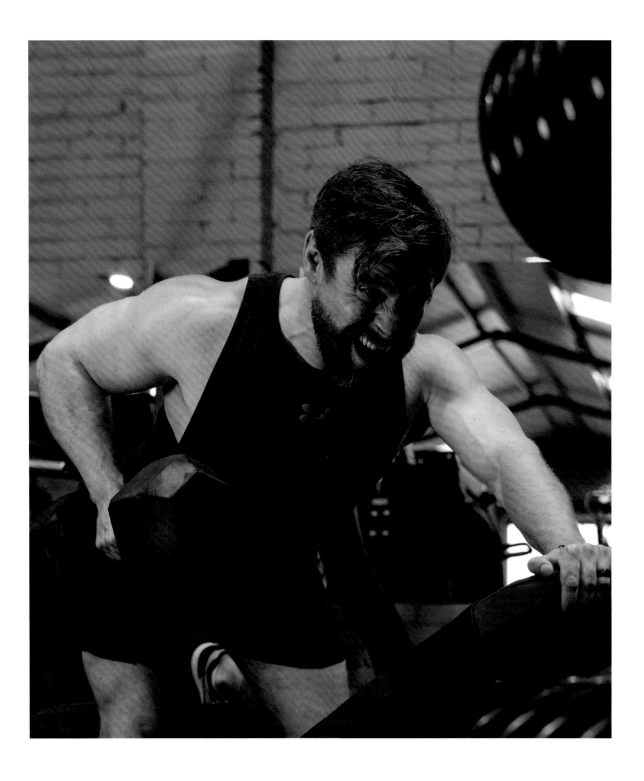

Having said that, some people think 'effort' means you need to be profusely sweating and red-faced, with veins popping out of your forehead. You don't have to turn into the Incredible Hulk to get results. You should, however, be pushing yourself to the point of struggle. If you're doing multiple sets of exercises, aim to use your first set as a bit of a warm-up, and then push yourself further on the second and third sets. There should come a point where you need to use some mental strength and focus, as well as physical effort, to get the job done. That's when you know you're putting in the kind of intensity that is required for change. I like to use this very simple rule of thumb: if you're starting to make involuntary noises out of sheer effort, you're probably using the correct amount of effort and weight.

Principle #3: Progressive overload

If you use the exact same weights for ever, you're not going to progress. Over time, your muscles will adapt and you'll build strength, which is great! But to continue to get results, you'll need to increase the weight. However, this progress should be incremental. Don't expect to add significant weight each time you go to the gym. Instead, look to nudge up the weight bit by bit.

To put this into perspective, I like to use a story about Milo of Croton, a Greek athlete from the sixth century BC. Milo was a famed wrestler, renowned for his remarkable strength. The story goes that Milo began as something of a weakling. One day, he noticed a calf had just been born on the farm. He picked up the wee calf, put it on his shoulders, and carried it around a while before returning it to its mother. The next day he came back to the calf and repeated the feat. He did this every single day, continuing even as the calf got older and bigger and eventually became a full-grown ox. Because Milo kept carrying the calf as it grew, he too grew stronger. By the time the calf was an ox, Milo had no problem carrying it around, showing off his impressive strength to the other villagers and his competition.

That story is the perfect parable for progressive overload. If you slowly and incrementally increase the weights you're lifting, in time, you will become stronger and able to lift more than you imagined.

This, by the way, was the same approach I took to improving my lung function post-hospitalisation. I knew that I couldn't snap my fingers and restore my lung function to 100 per cent. (I wish.) Instead, I focused on minute improvements. Each day, I would think to myself, *What could I do today to help my lung function improve by 1 per cent?* This took patience and dedication, but it worked. Eventually the doctors couldn't believe how much my lung function had improved. But I could believe it, because I had worked hard for each little improvement, day by day.

In a gym context, progressive overload is simple: slowly and gradually add weight to your exercises. Sometimes with my clients I'll sneak on an extra 1.25 kilos at a time without telling them. Because they think they're using the same weight, they don't even notice the change. When I later tell them they lifted more weight without even realising it, they start to get an inkling that they can do more than they've been giving themselves credit for. Of course, if you're working out solo you can't be quite this sneaky. But if you add just a tiny bit more than you're comfortable with, you might surprise yourself.

Principle #4: **Rest**

As you've learned throughout this book, recovery is just as important as effort. Balance your hard work – the stress you're putting on your body through exercise – with good recovery, and you'll improve. This is necessary within the gym as well. I'm all for making the most of your gym time, but if you try to race through your exercises with no rest, you're not going to be able to do your best work.

That's why you need to take some rest periods between your sets. This will help you get your breath back and help your muscles feel somewhat refreshed before working hard again. The time you take to rest will depend on the exercise, your current capacity and your energy levels that day. Large muscle groups like your legs and back will take a little longer to recover than smaller muscles like your shoulders or arms. Basically, the larger the muscle, the longer it will take to recover.

One caveat – don't fall into the trap of letting a quick break steal away your entire workout. You don't want to wind up on your phone answering emails or getting caught up in a lengthy conversation with a friend. You're there to exercise. Additionally, if you stop moving altogether for an extended period, your body can start to cool down, meaning you won't be as warmed up and primed for exercise, setting you up for potential injury.

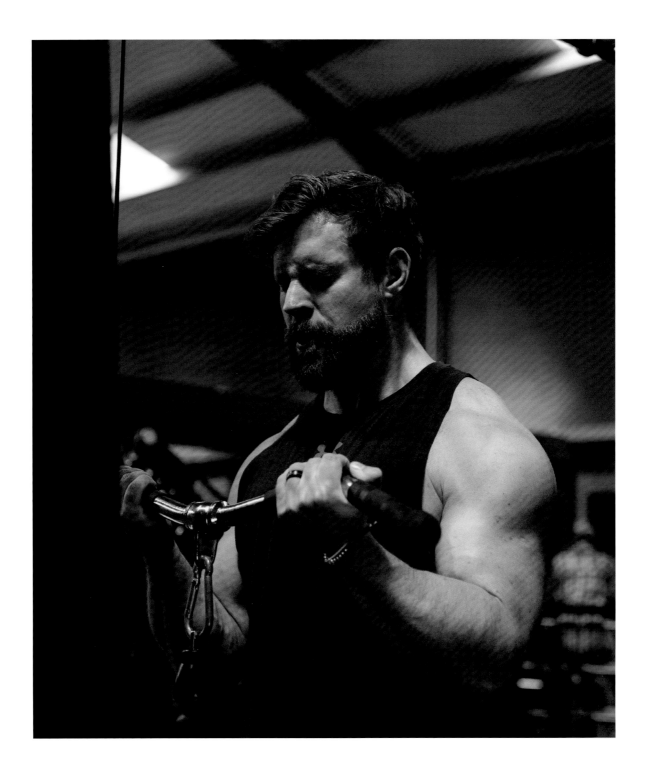

To make the most of your rest periods, I recommend setting a timer for two minutes. During that time you can walk around the gym and get in a few extra steps while letting your heart rate come down. Have a drink of water, take some deep breaths, and then return to the task at hand.

Principle #5: Tempo

Tempo refers to the rate, or speed, at which you move a weight during an exercise. In other words, how quickly you are pulling, pushing, squatting etc. That might not sound important (and it is at the top of my principles pyramid) but it can affect your movement quality, and whether you get results from your efforts.

Occasionally, I've seen people swinging weights around wildly in the gym. Think bicep curls being done super quickly, with lots of vacillating movement and momentum. These folks aren't keeping adequate tension on their muscles; instead, they're relying on momentum to get the weights up. This is a mistake. To get best results from your efforts, you must keep tension on your muscles. Challenge your muscles to move during tension, and they will get stronger.

Any lift should involve both eccentric (lengthening/stretching) movement, and concentric (shortening/contracting) movement of the muscle.

I like to think of this as 'Beauty and The Beast'. Imagine, for example, that you're doing a bicep curl. You start by holding the weight with a bent elbow, so the weight is close to your face. Next, while maintaining tension, you slowly lengthen your arm until your elbow is no longer bent. That lengthening is the 'Beauty' – it's an elegant, slow lengthening of the muscle. Your elbow, while bending, should otherwise remain locked in place throughout the movement. Next, you shorten the muscle by bringing your fist upwards and bending your elbow. Again, even as the elbow bends it should otherwise remain in place. This upwards movement should be faster and quicker. This movement is what I refer to as 'The Beast' – it's the tougher, quicker, more aggressive part of the movement.

Tempo can be tricky to master; it might not be immediately obvious to you which part of the movement is Beauty and which part is Beast, at least when you're starting out. If it helps, here's another way to think about it: load the

Load the movement, don't move the load.

movement, don't move the load. The goal isn't actually to move the load (i.e. the weight) from place to place. The point of a bicep curl isn't to get that weight higher in the air. The point of it is to be able to curl and uncurl your arm, while also holding a weight. It's the movement that matters.

A simple way to practise this is to concentrate on the movement itself. Pay attention to the muscles you want to target; see if you can feel them working. If you're doing a bicep curl, for example, pay attention to your bicep. Notice how it expands and contracts as you conduct the movement. The more you can notice and tap into your muscle exertion, the better and more natural your tempo will get – even for more complex exercises and muscles you're less familiar with.

(Note: I've used bicep curls as an example because most people know what they are. But most of the time, you won't be doing bicep curls – unless you very deliberately want to target them in addition to your standard workout. More often than not, you'll be doing compound movements, which I'll discuss shortly.)

Five myths about resistance training

Now that I've covered some principles of resistance training, some thoughts might start popping into your head like, 'but what about this thing I saw online' or 'but I read you have to do such and such'.

The internet in general, and the fitness industry in particular, can present a wealth of misinformation. It's easy to have preconceived notions or misunderstandings about what resistance training involves for the average person, and these ideas can get in your way or make things unnecessarily complicated.

If you're hesitant to try resistance training, or you're stuck on doing things a particular way, it could be that you've been misinformed. Let's lighten the load by clearing up some common myths.

Myth #1: **You need to focus on one muscle group per workout, as in 'leg day'**

You may have heard that you should structure your weightlifting/resistance training programme by muscle group. Using this method, sometimes called a 'bro split', you'd train legs and glutes one day, back muscles another day, arms and shoulders another day, abs another day.

I'll discuss 'splits' – a method of programming that involves splitting up muscle groups or movement types into different workouts – in the next section. For now, let me address this idea that workouts need to be oriented around one muscle or muscle group at a time.

Spoiler alert: you don't need to do it. Here's why.

The 'bro split' method comes from bodybuilders. And unless you *are* a bodybuilder, I suggest you don't train like one. Think about it: if you wanted to learn to drive a car, you wouldn't take driving lessons from a Formula One driver. The car and driving conditions they're used to are completely different from driving in everyday life.

Most professional bodybuilders have been building their muscles for over a decade. When your muscles are already well developed, you need to work that muscle more – put more stress on it – for it to continue to grow. That's why bodybuilders tend to split their workouts by muscle group. Their muscle tissue is that much stronger, so they need to put more stress on each muscle within a given workout to get results.

Most people don't need to train particular muscles that intensely for that long in a single workout. Suppose a typical exerciser does two or three sets of a leg press. That's enough to work that muscle adequately to initiate muscle growth or adaptation. For a bodybuilder, though, that's not necessarily going to do the trick, so they might do three sets of a leg press *and* three sets of squats *and* three sets of hamstring curls in one session.

Further, bodybuilders are being judged on the size and shape of their muscles, so many of them perform specific exercises to appeal to judging criteria.

Additionally, bodybuilders tend to spend *a lot* of time in the gym. When you're working out most days of the week, maybe even multiple workouts per day, you'll need a more complex programme to accommodate your schedule. The bottom line is that even if your goal is to get swole, you don't need to train like a bodybuilder. Forget the 'bro split' and plan your workout another way.

Myth #2: If you're not sore the next day, you didn't work hard enough

The following day or two after a workout, your muscles might feel tight and sore. This is something called Delayed Onset Muscle Soreness (or DOMS). If you've ever done a bunch of heavy squats or leg presses and then screamed in pain when getting off the toilet the next day, you're familiar with DOMS.

DOMS is caused by tiny tears in the muscle fibres that can occur during strenuous exercise such as weightlifting. This is a natural part of the process, and if you fuel your body properly (i.e. eat adequate protein and calories post-workout), your muscles should recover and grow bigger and stronger. However, while muscle soreness isn't a sign that something terrible is happening, it's also not essential for you to have a good workout.

Typically, DOMS occurs when a person is new to exercise, or does an exercise they don't have much experience with. For example, if you're a runner and you try powerlifting for the first time, you'll probably be sore the next day. And vice versa: a powerlifter who isn't used to running will probably be sore too. Luckily, as time passes and your body becomes more acclimatised to a particular exercise, you'll likely experience less muscle soreness. This doesn't mean your body isn't still adapting – if you're doing challenging workouts and recovering well, you will continue to get stronger and develop your muscles.

Yet, perhaps because of the old 'no pain, no gain' attitude, some people equate soreness with a successful workout. But a lot of soreness isn't ideal; in fact, it can inhibit your overall results. If you're super sore, how likely are you to sneak in extra movement? Are you going to park your car further away from your office? Are you going to take the stairs rather than the elevator? Probably not. It's more likely you'll avoid moving because it hurts! That means you won't be able to take full advantage of NEAT, the benefits of which I discussed in Part One, and you'll decrease your movement overall.

Furthermore, while it's natural for beginners to feel sore, lasting pain can be a sign that you're not recovering properly. As I've said, with adequate protein, calories and rest, your body shouldn't be too sore – at least not for long. This doesn't mean soreness is bad, but the goal should be to bounce back quickly from your workouts so you can carry on with being active and feel good for your next workout.

I go by the motto, 'stimulate, don't annihilate'. Yes, you want to challenge your muscles (and yourself). That's how you'll get results. But challenging yourself doesn't mean you need to overdo it. Recovering well is a sign you're doing things right.

Myth #3: The best way to train is . . . [enter workout routine here]

If you're wondering 'What's the best workout plan?', I have an answer for you. The best workout plan or programme is the one that works for *you*. It's one that you enjoy, and one you can stick to.

That answer might sound like a bit of a cop-out, but the truth is that everybody and every *body* is different. Exercise is suitable for everyone and yet no one in particular. General recommendations are meant to be adapted to specific circumstances.

Here's an example. A friend of mine is roughly the same height as me, but his proportions are very different. His arms and legs are longer and his torso is shorter, whereas my torso is longer and my arms and legs are shorter. With his long wingspan, bench pressing isn't ideal – his arms have much longer to go in order to reach his chest and push the weight away from his body, which means the movement isn't all that economical. More effort is needed for him to move the weight. I'm the opposite: my arms are shorter, which is a handy advantage in bench pressing. There's less distance required for me to get the weight down to my chest and back to the bar.

On the other hand, my friend is a great deadlifter. But for whatever reason, deadlifting has never quite agreed with me. I always wind up hurting my back, no matter how hard I work on getting my form just right. And before any hardcore deadlifting fans line up to tell me how to correct my form, my point is simply that you don't have to do any single particular exercise, let alone follow a particular plan or programme, in order to get results.

On that note, just as you don't need to follow someone else's method, nor do you need to subscribe to some new-fangled exercise system to get all the benefits of resistance training. The truth is that effective exercise isn't all that sexy. A lot of workout routines and systems are just fancied-up versions of the basics. People come up with clever names and systems, because it's easier to sell something that seems interesting and exciting than the same old basics. But the basics work.

Myth #4: Machines won't give you a 'real' workout

Machines aren't 'cool' these days. Admittedly, they're not as sexy as loading up a barbell with a bunch of weights, but if you're a beginner, machines are your friend.

My first foray into resistance training was a 'multigym' machine – one of those at-home gym machines that had all kinds of movements built into it. Before I ever set foot in a gym I learned the basics on that machine. That's how I went from a scrawny kid to a guy with some actual muscle. And it's how I started getting comfortable with some of the basic movements that are essential for moving well and developing a strong body, which I'll detail momentarily.

In case you need more convincing, here are some of the reasons why I'm a fan of workout machines, especially for beginners.

They teach you the proper movement

Because most of the machines you'll find in the gym are designed for a very particular movement, they tend to prevent you from doing things incorrectly. For example, if you learn how to do a chest press on a machine, you'll likely find it much easier to perform the movement correctly when using a barbell or dumbbells.

They're safe

Have you ever done a bench press with no spotter, and found yourself lying back on the bench, squashed under a bar loaded with heavy weights and unable to move? I have. Trust me, it's a humbling experience and one you're better off avoiding. Machines are designed to prevent mistakes, which makes them great for beginners.

They tend to accommodate higher reps, giving you more practice

Machines are somewhat assisted, making them a bit 'easier'. And while you can always load up the weight, doing movements at a lower weight but for more reps is advantageous when you're just starting out. It gives you more practice repeating a movement, so it becomes more ingrained. (There's that principle of Frequency at work!)

They're somewhat private

Depending on their construction and how they're situated in the gym, machines tend to give you a little bit of privacy. It can feel daunting for newbies to take up space among the free weights or at a squat rack. While I want you to get past the intimidation factor eventually, there's nothing wrong with starting where you feel more comfortable. Build up your confidence a bit before taking centre stage on the lifting platform.

They're efficient

For people who have limited time, machines can make the whole process go quicker. After all, loading up a bar takes time. Case in point: for a while, hip thrusts were a big part of my routine. Because I'm pretty experienced, I needed quite a lot of weight on the bar. That meant I had to use thin – but heavy – weight plates, which were located across the gym. I had to walk across the gym, back and forth, carrying the weight plates and loading them onto the bar just to do my hip thrusts. This became a workout in itself! Plus, I think people were starting to wonder about the weirdo who kept carrying plates back and forth through the gym. Eventually I stopped bothering with the bar and moved to a hip-thrust machine where I could easily add adequate weight and get the sets done.

This is not to say you need to use machines – of course you don't. I'll show you movements you can do a variety of ways. But depending on your experience and what you need from your workout, they can be an asset.

Myth #5: When it comes to your workouts, you need to go big or go home

'Fitness content' – or 'fitspo' – tends to emphasise themes like 'beast mode', 'kicking ass' or 'go big or go home'. That's fine if it inspires you. But in real life, 'beast mode' is pretty rare. Most of the time, you'll probably find yourself in 'just doing my best to get it done mode' or 'squeezing in a workout between a hectic workday and making dinner for the kids mode'.

Realistically, in ten gym sessions, one or two will be fantastic, two or three will suck, and the rest will be okay. Bad sessions are inevitable. (Just as inevitable as me buying way too much Warhammer.) Some days you might be tired, stressed, sore or strapped for time. The gym might be full of annoying people, or playing the wrong type of music. Some days you'll just be going through the motions and getting it done. On the other hand, some days you'll be at your peak, full of energy and ready to reach a personal best. All of these are perfectly acceptable. Bad sessions are just as much part of this process as good ones. If you keep coming back and showing up regardless of how you feel, the results will come.

Amrita: From exercise machines to the squat rack

If you have any doubt as to whether workout machines are worth using, or whether you deserve a place among the hardcore gym lifters, consider my client Amrita.

At fifty-five years old, Amrita had no experience with formal exercise. Simply walking into the gym meant she was getting out of her comfort zone. To help her start out on the right foot, I designed a programme for her that used the machines her gym had to offer. Following my programme, she was able to practise various movements to build her strength and confidence.

After six months using the machines, Amrita told me she was ready to expand her comfort zone and push herself a bit more. I suggested she try replacing her machine leg press with a goblet squat, using a dumbbell. She agreed, but I noticed some hesitation.

When I asked her about it, she admitted that she felt intimidated by the free weight area. 'It feels like the "guys" section,' she said.

While that term made me cringe – it's definitely not just for 'guys' – I could empathise with Amrita. Yes, I'm a guy. But in my early days, I used to feel like that section was reserved for the big, bro-y muscle dudes. Remember, when I first started working out, I was a small guy, and a total novice to boot.

'First off,' I said to Amrita, 'I get it. I've been a beginner myself. But everyone starts out as a beginner. We were all new to this at some point.

'Besides,' I added, 'that is not the "guys" area. It's *your* area. It belongs to everyone and anyone. You pay just as much as them for a gym membership, so you have every right to work out there.'

Amrita took in what I was saying. 'Okay, Ben,' she said. 'I want to get out of my comfort zone anyway. It's time.'

I taught Amrita how to do a goblet squat and made sure she was prepared. The next week, she walked up to the rack, grabbed a dumbbell, and did her very first goblet squats.

Amrita completed her set with a sense of pride. And she was pleasantly surprised. Far from being critical or snobby, a few of the guys applauded her effort and commented that she had great form.

Since then, Amrita has been a regular in the lifting area of her gym. She still uses some machines for her accessory work, but she can often be found doing squats, bench presses and deadlifts with total confidence. I have no doubt that, as well as impressing herself, she's inspiring others.

SECTION B: STRUCTURING YOUR WORKOUTS

Now that I've covered some basics – and cleared up some misconceptions – let's consider the 'how' of resistance training. In this section, I'll introduce compound movements, explain three types of workouts you can consider, and give you a fun idea to make your workouts most efficient and impactful.

Compound movements

While the body can move in lots of different ways, there are some core movements that are very useful for functional, 'real life' strength. These are fundamental, 'bread and butter' movements that can be trained in a multitude of ways, and I typically include them in some shape or form in all my clients' programmes.

Most of these movements are compound movements, meaning they involve several joints at the same time. A single exercise that involves multiple joints, like a barbell squat, will deliver more benefit than a single exercise that involves just one, like a leg extension, which expressly targets the thighs/quads.

I like to use the following analogy to explain the difference between compound movements and isolation movements (which isolate just one muscle). Think of isolation movements and compound movements like

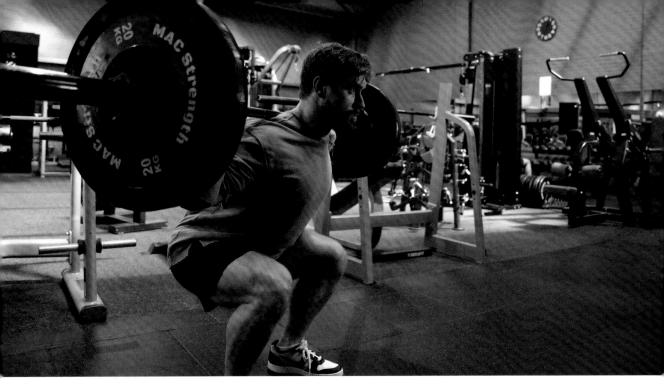

race cars and rally cars respectively. A Formula One race car is designed perfectly to do one task: drive really fast around the track. Similarly, isolation movements are designed to focus on just one muscle at a time, making them suitable for bodybuilding. Rally cars, on the other hand, are agile and versatile, capable of more diverse kinds of driving. Compound movements are similar, making them a good option for most people. Both movements have their place, but for general training, compound exercises tend to be more practical.

In Part Three, I'll show you which compound movements are best to focus on, and how to do them.

Types of workouts

There are endless ways to put together a resistance training programme, but to keep things simple, here are three options to consider. As you'll see, the first one – the full body workout – is broadly applicable and will work for the majority of people reading this book. However, I've provided two more options for those want to mix things up.

The three options are:

- **Full body**
- **Upper-lower**
- **Push-pull-legs**

Full body

What it is: Just as it sounds, a full body workout involves the entire body, rather than working specific muscle groups. It can make great use of the compound movements you just learned about. Typically, a full body workout will train muscle groups such as your back, your chest, your arms, your core (including your abs) and your legs.

Who it's best suited for: Beginners; people with active hobbies (such as football or long-distance running); people who are able to train one to three days per week.

Benefits: It is hands down the most flexible and accessible type of workout. It has many benefits:

- It allows you to work your whole body within a given session, making it both efficient and effective.

- It's typically performed with a full day off in between (e.g. Mondays, Wednesdays and Fridays). This gives you time to recover and enjoy other active hobbies or sports.

- Since you're working your whole body, rather than overtaxing a single muscle group, you'll have more energy in between sessions, supporting general movement and fat loss.

- It's highly adaptable. You can adjust your workouts based on your schedule, your energy level and your resources (i.e. what weights you have available to you).

- It can be more enjoyable because you're not working any particular muscles into the ground.

Upper-lower

What it is: An upper-lower workout is a form of workout known as a 'split', which basically means you break up your workouts to target different muscles over the course of a week or two. As you might imagine, the upper-lower split breaks your workouts into two groups: the upper body and the lower body. Upper body includes your back, chest, shoulders, arms and core (including abs). Lower body includes glutes (your bum muscles), hamstrings, quads and calves.

Who it's best suited for: People who have been training consistently three times per week for a minimum of twelve weeks who want to add more volume, such as four workouts per week. People who are seeking muscle growth but already have well-developed muscles and want to target certain muscle groups more deliberately.

Benefits: The upper-lower split allows you to exercise a bit more frequently (such as four days per week) while still recovering adequately. While you wouldn't want to do two or more full body workouts back-to-back, you can get away with this by working your upper body one day and your lower body the next (or vice versa).

Another potential benefit to the upper-lower split, if you are an experienced exerciser, is that it will allow you to target specific muscles a bit more intensively. Well-developed muscles can require more stress to break down and grow. A split can enable you to do that, since you're devoting entire workouts to one region of the body.

Push-pull-legs

What it is: This type of workout is another form of split. In this case, the workouts are divided into three groups: upper-body 'pushing' muscles, upper-body 'pulling' muscles and legs.

- Your pushing muscles typically include your triceps, shoulders and chest.
- Your pulling muscles would involve your back, biceps and rear delts.
- Legs, as you might guess, includes your leg muscles such as your quads, hamstrings, calves and glutes.

(By the way, don't worry if you don't know all the anatomical terminology just yet. I'll break everything down for you in the next part of the book.)

You'll engage your core muscles naturally while doing this type of workout, but if you'd like to specifically target your core or abdomen, you could tack on some core work as well.

Who it's best suited for: People who have been training consistently for one or more years, and who want to train more frequently and/or increase the volume of work.

Benefits: This type of workout is similar to an upper-lower split, but it allows you to increase the volume of work on certain muscle groups while still getting adequate rest between workouts. For example, say you're doing four exercises per workout. If you're doing a full body workout, you need to do exercises that target muscles throughout the body. But if you're just working your pulling muscles, you can give your back, biceps and delts a pretty good workout. In slightly more technical terms, this means you can increase the volume of work, but because you're spreading the workouts over different muscle groups, you can still get forty-eight hours of rest before working those muscles again. Personally, I enjoy training this way – and enjoyment is a key factor. Once again, this type of workout isn't necessarily better than the others, it's just another option.

The bottom line

For the vast amount of people – and certainly beginners – I would recommend starting with full body workouts. Don't let the other options confuse or overwhelm you. It's perfectly acceptable to keep your workouts simple without complicating things with workout splits.

That said, I don't want you to be limited by your training options. There are many styles out there. As you get increasingly comfortable and confident in the gym, you can explore different types of programmes.

What about home workouts or bodyweight exercises?

Workouts using simple equipment, such as resistance bands or bodyweight only, can be effective, especially when your options are limited – as they were during the COVID-19 pandemic, when gyms were closed and people were confined to their homes. However, if possible, I encourage people to get to the gym and give lifting weights a try.

There are a few reasons for this. For one thing, it will be easier to get more and better results when you're lifting actual weights. It's like using a hand screwdriver vs a power screwdriver. The hand screwdriver can do the job, but it's going to be a lot slower and more difficult.

The other reason for this is that going to the gym can help you build confidence and get out of your comfort zone. The more you push against your comfort zone, the more it expands. If going to the gym makes you nervous, embrace it. Know that by continually showing up, you're challenging that self-doubt and building your internal confidence. This is necessary to break out of your perceived limitations.

Furthermore, when you go to the gym, you're entering a space in which you can purely focus on yourself. If you're working out at home, chances are there are other people and distractions around. Your kids want your attention, the dog wants to be walked, the dirty dishes in the kitchen are begging to be washed. When you're in the gym, you can take some time just for you.

I understand that people have busy lives and often feel like they can't take time away just for themselves, but I promise you, if you can find a way to swing it, everyone and everything else will still be there when you get back.

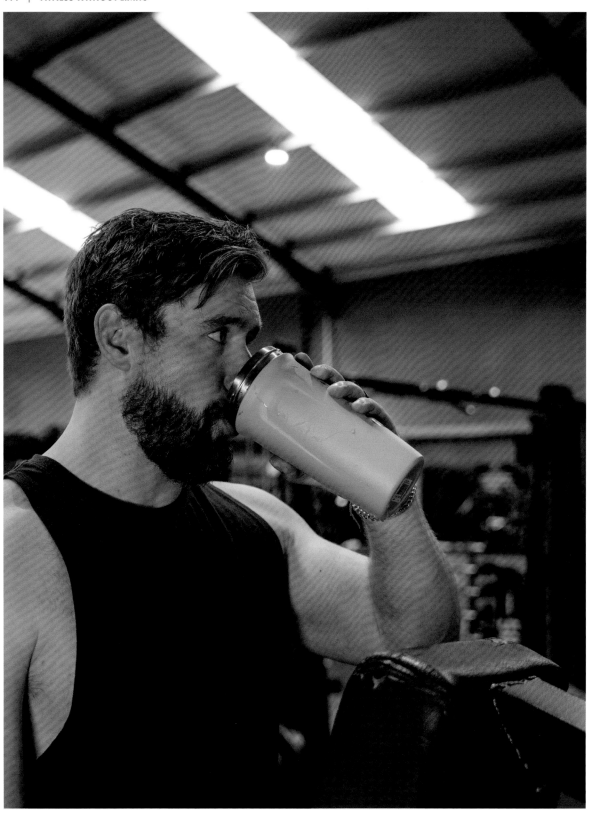

Two workout components: Main Mission and Side Quest

Now that you've learned about workout types, here's how to put different exercises together into a programme or routine. In Part Three, I'll share specific exercises you can choose from. For now, think of this as general guidance as to how you might conceptualise your workouts.

A solid workout typically involves two components. Maybe it's the nerd in me, but rather than think about primary and secondary components (boring), I like to think of these as your 'Main Mission' and your 'Side Quest'. It's more fun to imagine yourself as a hero beginning an epic adventure, rather than just another person in the gym.

- Your **Main Mission** (or primary component) will tackle your big muscle groups and involve compound movements. (As a reminder, compound movements target multiple muscles and multiple joints at once.)
- The **Side Quest** (or secondary component) will target smaller muscle groups, such as shoulders, biceps or triceps. This can be useful if there are specific muscles you want to target – for example if you want more defined calves or more visible abs. This is where you might use a mix of isolation and compound movements.

If you have a full hour to exercise, you can probably fit in both your Main Mission and Side Quest. But if time is scarce – say you have forty-five minutes or less – you can choose to prioritise your Main Mission. While both workouts are useful, your Main Mission will address more muscle groups, delivering the most value for your time. Plus, you'll still be stimulating those smaller muscles. The muscles in your shoulders and arms will still be engaged when you perform a deadlift, they're just not working as hard as the muscles in, say, your legs and glutes. That said, the Side Quest can still be useful – it can help you focus on smaller muscles that might not otherwise get as much attention. But it's more of a 'nice to have'.

I'll show you exactly what to do in your Main Mission and Side Quest in Part Three.

SECTION C: SCHEDULING AND SUPPORTING YOUR PROGRAMME

In this section, I'll discuss how often you should work out, how to make the most of your rest days and other activities, and how to build an exercise schedule that works for you. Let's begin with scheduling.

Scheduling your workouts

When it comes to scheduling, the first question to consider is how often you want to train each week.

To figure this out, you need to consider two things. First, how often do you *want* to work out? And second, how often *can* you work out?

Your frequency will depend on these two things. There's no point committing to a schedule that you can't maintain. Why strive for four workouts a week when only two workouts are possible?

For example, suppose in an ideal world, you want to hit the gym four times a week, but you know that in busy weeks, only two sessions will be possible. In that case, make two sessions your baseline and consider anything more than that a bonus. In weeks when you have more time, hit the gym as much as you want! Go ahead and work out four times if you can. But know that if you've been twice, that's good enough.

Your ability to make progress depends on your ability to recover.

If your expectations for yourself are too high, you'll wind up feeling defeated or as if your best effort wasn't good enough. On the other hand, if you wind up doing more than expected, you'll feel like you're crushing it and you'll be more motivated and encouraged to keep going. Human psychology is a funny thing, but we can use it to our advantage by keeping our expectations fair and realistic.

If all else fails, remember that something is always better than nothing. A client recently said to me, 'I can only get to the gym once a week at this point. I've tried to make time for additional workouts but it's just not happening.' In response, I asked him, 'Is one session not a hundred per cent better than zero?' Remember that if you ever think you're not doing enough.

Once you know how often you're prepared to train each week, you can move on to creating a workout schedule for yourself. When scheduling, you'll want to plan not only your workouts but also your rest days, or more accurately, something called 'active recovery'.

Scheduling your active recovery

The importance of recovery cannot be underestimated. Your ability to recover will have a significant impact on your ability to proceed with your workouts and all other undertakings. As you learned back in Principle #1 about sleep, your recovery should be equal to or greater than the stress you're putting on your body – which includes exercise. That means, no matter how much you're working out, you need to support your body's ability to recover by resting, sleeping, eating well and managing the other stressors in your life. Trust me on this: your ability to make progress depends on your ability to recover.

To bring this idea together, imagine you're sitting in a rowing boat with two oars. Your training represents one oar; your recovery represents the other. Both oars are of equal importance. If you only use one oar, you'll just be going around in circles. But use both equally and you'll surely make progress.

Ideally, to get adequate recovery you'll want to give your body a full forty-eight hours between workouts. This is especially true if you're doing a full body workout. If you're doing a split, such as upper-lower, then you have a bit more flexibility, because you're not targeting all of your muscle groups within the same workout. While your legs will still get a bit of a workout during an upper body workout, they'll be pretty fresh and ready to move the next day. That said, you'll still want to schedule recovery days throughout the week; don't do more than two splits back-to-back if you can avoid it.

Notably, recovery doesn't mean lying on the couch all day. In fact, some medium-intensity movement can help you recover by encouraging blood flow and decreasing muscle soreness. That's why I encourage active recovery. That said, if you feel like you need a full rest, take it. And if you generally feel so worn out by your workouts that you don't have energy for active recovery, dial things back – that's a sign you're pushing too much.

In Part Three, I'll show you exactly how to put your workouts together and provide some sample schedules that incorporate both exercise sessions and active recovery.

What is active recovery?

Active recovery involves light to moderate movement that supports your body in the recovery process and helps it to bounce back after workouts. I recommend seeking out activities that you find enjoyable and/or stress-relieving.

Some ideas: playing sports with friends, going for walks or hikes (take the dog with you if you have one!), swimming, cycling, jogging, climbing, doing yoga, dancing, gardening, kayaking, stand-up paddle-boarding, playing with your kids in the park . . . the list goes on.

All these things count as active recovery and can be excellent sources of movement to help your body – and mind – recover from not only your workouts, but all of life's stresses. Plus, as you've learned, they contribute to your NEAT, helping you burn calories and supporting your general health.

Summary

We've covered a lot in this part of the book! To recap, we've explored the basics of resistance training, how to structure your workouts, and how to schedule and support your workout programme.

If there's one thing I want you to take away from this part, it's to get yourself into the gym and give resistance training a try. If you're a beginner, learning your way around the gym might feel uncomfortable at first, but it's worth it. Challenge yourself, nudge yourself out of your comfort zone, and little by little you'll start to see how incredibly capable you are.

Exercising, and resistance training in particular, can be incredibly rewarding. You'll get to see your strength develop before your very eyes as weights or movements that once seemed incredibly difficult become almost too easy. Better still, exercising *in* the gym is a gateway to thriving *out* of the gym. It's a way to cast off your limitations and discover a whole new world of possibilities for yourself.

Your workouts don't have to be mind-blowingly fantastic, nor do you have to enter full-blown 'beast mode' to benefit from them. Show up, give it your best effort, repeat – and the results will come.

 RECAP

Resistance training essentials:

- Choose your workout type (full body, upper-lower split or push-pull-legs split)

- Choose your Main Mission and Side Quest

- Schedule your workout (one to four days per week)

- Schedule your active recovery (do some light to moderate activity on your non-workout days)

- Follow the key principles of resistance training:

  1. Frequency
  2. Intensity
  3. Progressive overload
  4. Rest
  5. Tempo

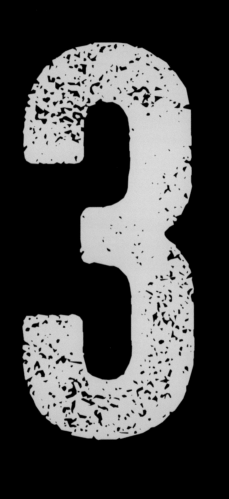

PART THREE

PROGRAMME DESIGNER

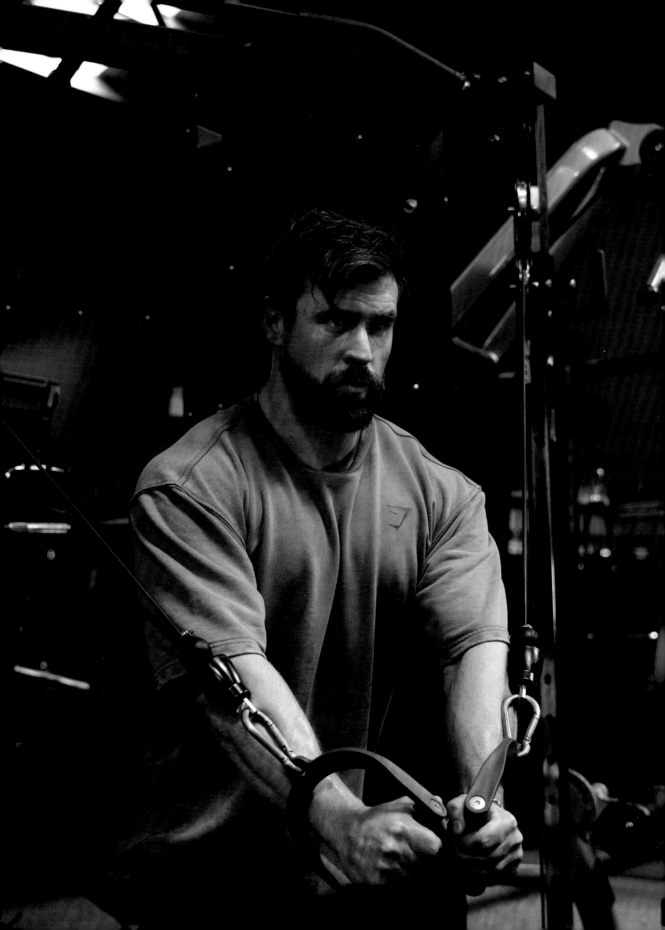

Exercise programming has the potential to be very complex and detailed. My goal here is to do the opposite and keep things as simple as possible.

Let's get back to basics

Resistance training doesn't have to be complicated to deliver results. In fact, the simpler you make things for yourself, the more likely you'll be able to master the basics, keep showing up, and reap the benefits.

In this part of the book I'll provide you with a simple 'programme designer' – a tool for you to create effective yet relatively straightforward workouts for yourself. This programme designer works like a 'pick and mix': You can choose from the options depending on your familiarity with exercise, your own preferences and the equipment you have available.

First, I'll guide you through the process of building your own workout. Then I'll take you through my 'exercise menu' and show you how everything works. By the end, you'll have a very simple system for choosing exercises, and when you go to the gym you'll know exactly what to do.

HOW TO BUILD YOUR OWN WORKOUT

To build your own workout, choose four of the following movements: a squat, a hinge, a lunge, a pull, a push, or a core exercise.

I've selected these particular movements because they provide the foundation of good movement, strength and mobility. Most people can do them and they don't require a complex set-up – you can find ways of doing them using dumbbells, barbells or the most basic of machines. Plus, if you're interested in such things, they happen to make the body look nice and strong too.

When you can comfortably and confidently do these kinds of movements – squatting, pushing, pulling, lunging, hinging and engaging your core – you are going to be better able to meet the challenges and opportunities of life. You can push your kids on a swing or carry them when they claim they're too tired to walk home from the park. You can move your sofa to vacuum underneath it or rearrange the furniture of your house without hurting your back. You can hike up a mountain . . . or just bend over and tie your shoes with ease. You can get up and off a toilet seat, which might sound like nothing now, but can be the difference between independence and requiring constant care when you're elderly.

The exercises I've suggested will also enable you to keep your workouts short and sweet, so you can get out of the gym and back to living your life. For the most part, they involve compound movements which, as you've now learned, engage multiple muscle groups at a time. These compound movements in particular target the main muscle groups in the body, which means they're your best way to get fit.

With all that in mind, here's how to choose your exercises from the menu of options and put everything together in a sequence that works for you. As you read on, you'll see options for adapting these to full body workouts, or various splits.

Step 1. Choose your workout type

In Part Two, I outlined three different workout options, or 'training splits':

- Full body
- Upper-lower
- **Push-pull-legs**

To choose which one will work best for you, start by deciding how many days a week you can realistically train. Base this on your busiest week, not your ideal week.

Do you expect to train twice per week? A full body workout split will probably be your best option as it will allow you to target all the major muscle groups in one session.

If you plan to train three or four times per week, I suggest an upper-lower split. (Though a full body workout would be fine too.)

If your schedule allows you to train five times a week, push-pull-legs might work best. (Though upper-lower is an option there as well.)

Training days per week	Recommended training split
1–2	Full body
3–4	Upper-lower (or full body)
4+	Push-pull-legs (or upper-lower)

One added consideration is experience level. The more lifting experience you have, the more training volume you'll need in order to see growth. In this case, it may help you to try new training splits. In general, I recommend full body workouts for beginners; intermediate lifters may want to try upper-lower splits, and advanced lifters may want to try either upper-lower or push-pull-leg splits.

Training level	Recommended training split
Beginner	Full body
Intermediate	Full body or upper-lower
Advanced	Upper-lower or push-pull-legs

Bottom line: aim to select a training split that works best for your training level and your availability. Remember, you can always adjust as you go.

Step 2. Choose your Main Mission and (optionally) your Side Quest

To create a simple and efficient workout, simply pick four exercises from the exercise menu on page 160. The four exercises you choose are your Main Mission. As you've learned, this is your basic workout. You don't need to do anything more than four exercises per workout.

Why four exercises? I like to aim for four because it gives you a good mix of the essential movements while keeping things simple. Psychologically, it's pretty easy to commit to just four exercises. This gives you a workout that is efficient, effective and achievable.

Here's what this can look like in practice. Suppose you're doing a full body workout, and you want to do a squat, a hinge, a push and a pull. For each of these movements, you'll choose one exercise that corresponds with this movement (e.g., a goblet squat, a deadlift, a bench press and a pull-up).

If you have the luxury of a bit more time or some extra energy, you can add two more exercises to the mix – this is your Side Quest. If you're doing both a Main Mission and a Side Quest, that means you'll do six different movements.

Step 3. Choose your difficulty level

For each movement, I've given you a few exercise options, ranging in difficulty level from one to three.

The higher difficulty levels signify exercises that are more fatiguing and/or a bit more complex. For example, a barbell back squat is a higher difficulty level not just because it's a physically challenging exercise, but also because it demands a bit more refinement in terms of body position and muscle engagement. On the other hand, a dumbbell goblet squat (where you squat while holding a dumbbell in your hands as if it's a goblet) is more straightforward.

When in doubt, choose the exercises that feel most doable and understandable to you. I don't want you exerting a lot of mental energy trying to figure out how to do something. It's perfectly okay – even advantageous – to stick with exercises that feel more comfortable and intuitive to you.

However, if you do want to challenge yourself, you can try adding a couple of the more difficult exercises here and there. Sprinkle them in, rather than jumping an entire level all at once. If you start out with mostly Level 1 exercises, try adding one or two Level 2 exercises to your next workout and get comfortable with them before continuing to upgrade.

Downgrading difficulty level is also a great option if you're tired or not feeling your best. If you're an intermediate exerciser and you typically use Level 2 or Level 3 exercises, you can use Level 1 exercises for days when you feel stressed or tired or have low energy.

Step 4. Choose your sequence

Wondering what order you should do your exercises in? Follow this simple rule of thumb: do the hardest, most fatiguing exercises first.

Think of your energy like an orange. When you first start squeezing the orange, you have the most juice. The more you squeeze out of the orange, the less juice you get and the harder you have to squeeze.

Some of your exercises will require more juice, so you'll want to do them at the beginning of the workout. If you are doing some Level 2 or Level 3 exercises, put them first in your exercise sequence. If all your exercises are the same difficulty level, I'd recommend putting your squat or hinge at the beginning of your workout since they tend to target larger muscle groups which can require more energy. If you're not doing a squat or hinge, put the push and pull first.

Step 5. Choose your number of reps and sets

Workouts are broken up by 'reps' and 'sets'.

Reps refer to how many repetitions of an exercise you do at a time.

Sets refer to how many rounds of an exercise you do. In other words, each time you do 8–12 squat reps, that counts as a set. Once you complete a set, move on to the next exercise.

To keep things simple, I recommend doing between one and four sets of 8–12 reps. For example, if you're doing squats, deadlifts, bench presses and pull-ups, do 8–12 squats, then 8–12 deadlifts, then 8–12 bench presses, then 8–12 pull-ups. Once you've completed one set of each exercise, rest for a couple of minutes. Then, if you're doing more than one set, repeat the entire circuit. Most of the time, 2–3 sets will work well. If you have a bit more time, feel good and want to push yourself, a fourth set is always an option. Then again, one set is perfectly acceptable too! If one set of your Main Mission is all you've got time for, no problem. Work with what you've got that day.

I would recommend taking at _least_ sixty seconds of rest between sets. If you are still tired you can increase the rest period up to two minutes. If you are a beginner, I would suggest taking longer breaks to ensure you are fresh for each set.

Step 6. Get it done

That's it. Now that you know what you're doing, all that's left is to jump in and get it done. And, in case you need another reminder, your best is good

*Some of your workouts are going to be killer.
But other times, you're going to feel like you're just
going through the motions. That's okay.*

enough! Getting to the gym is the hardest part. Now that you're here, all you need to do is complete your workout to the best of your abilities with the time that you've got.

Some of your workouts are going to be killer. But other times, you're going to feel like you're just going through the motions. That's okay. Scale things back if you need to. It's better to have a bunch of mediocre workouts than just one great one. Consistency matters.

If you don't enjoy your workouts at first, trust that they will get easier with time. Keep showing up and in time you'll feel a growing sense of satisfaction and pride in your efforts.

EXERCISE MENU

To build a workout, choose 4–6 movements from the options below. For each movement, choose a corresponding exercise from the following list.

Full body movement options

	Squat
	Hinge
	Lunge
	Pull
	Push
	Core

Upper-lower and push-pull-legs movement options

	Squat
	Hinge
	Lunge
	Pull
	Push
	Core
	Accessory

Equipment key

BB = Barbell

DB = Dumbbell

Mac = Machine

CBL = Cable

MB = Medicine ball

N/A = No equipment required

Exercise options

Squat

Exercise name	Equipment	Muscles used	Difficulty
Back squat	BB	Glutes, Hamstrings, Quads	3
Goblet squat	DB	Glutes, Hamstrings, Quads	1
Suitcase squat	DB	Glutes, Hamstrings, Quads	2
Smith machine squat	Mac	Glutes, Hamstrings, Quads	1
Hack squat	Mac	Glutes, Hamstrings, Quads	2
Split squat	DB	BB	Glutes, Hamstrings, Quads	3
Leg press	Mac	Glutes, Hamstrings, Quads	1

Hinge

Exercise name	Equipment	Muscles used	Difficulty
Deadlift	BB	Glutes, Erectors, Hamstrings, Lats	3
Trap bar deadlift	BB	Glutes, Erectors, Hamstrings, Lats	2
Sumo deadlift	BB	Glutes, Erectors, Hamstrings, Lats	2
Back extension	Mac	Glutes, Erectors	1
Hip thrust	BB	Mac	Glutes, Hamstrings	1
Romanian deadlift	BB	Glutes, Hamstrings	2

Lunge

Exercise name	Equipment	Muscles used	Difficulty
Static lunge	DB	BB	Quads, Hamstrings, Glutes, Calves	1
Walking lunge	DB	BB	Quads, Hamstrings, Glutes, Calves	2
Reverse lunge	DB	BB	Quads, Hamstrings, Glutes, Calves	3
Front elevated lunge	DB	BB	Quads, Hamstrings, Glutes, Calves	1
Lateral lunge	DB	BB	Quads, Hamstrings, Glutes, Calves	3
Step-up	DB	BB	Quads, Hamstrings, Glutes, Calves	1

Pull

Pull	Exercise name	Equipment	Muscles used	Difficulty
Vertical	Assisted pull-up	Mac	Lats, Delts, Biceps, Forearms	1
Vertical	Lat pulldown	Mac	Lats, Delts, Biceps, Forearms	1
Vertical	Neutral grip pulldown	Mac | CBL	Lats, Delts, Biceps, Forearms	1
Vertical	One arm pulldown	Mac | CBL	Lats, Delts, Biceps, Forearms	2
Vertical	Supinated pulldown	Mac | CBL	Lats, Delts, Biceps, Forearms	2
Vertical	Pull-up	N/A	Lats, Delts, Biceps, Forearms	3
Vertical	Chin-up	N/A	Lats, Delts, Biceps, Forearms	3
Horizontal	Seated row	Mac | CBL	Lats, Delts, Biceps, Forearms	1
Horizontal	Single arm row	Mac | CBL | DB	Lats, Delts, Biceps, Forearms	2
Horizontal	Bent over row	CBL | DB | BB	Lats, Delts, Biceps, Forearms, Erectors	1
Horizontal	Supinated row	CBL | DB	Lats, Delts, Biceps, Forearms	2
Horizontal	Inverted row	BB	Lats, Delts, Biceps, Forearms	3
Horizontal	T-bar row	Mac	Lats, Delts, Erectors, Biceps, Forearms	1

Push

Exercise name	Equipment	Muscles used	Difficulty
Bench press	DB | BB	Pecs, Delts, Triceps	2
Incline bench press	DB | BB | Mac | CBL	Pecs, Delts, Triceps	2
Chest press	Mac | CBL	Pecs, Delts, Triceps	1
Assisted dip	Mac	Pecs, Delts, Triceps	1
Dip	Mac	Pecs, Delts, Triceps	2
Shoulder press	DB | BB | Mac	Delts, Triceps	1
Single arm shoulder press	DB	Delts, Triceps	2

Core

Exercise name	Equipment	Muscles used	Difficulty
Suitcase carry	DB	Obliques, Abs	1
Medicine ball slam	MB	Abs	1
Medicine ball side slam	MB	Obliques, Abs	1
Bicycle crunch	N/A	Obliques, Abs	1
Deadbug	N/A	Obliques, Abs	1
Bird dog	N/A	Obliques, Abs	1
Crunch	N/A	Abs	1

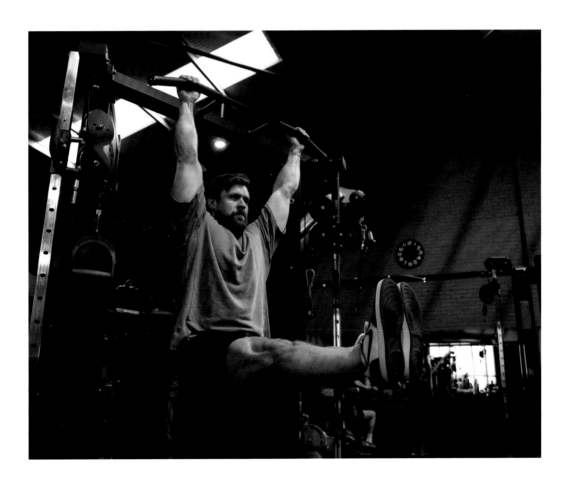

Additional Side Quest options for upper-lower splits

If doing an upper-lower split, you may choose to incorporate some additional Side Quest exercises from the following options.

Accessory exercises for 'upper' workout

Accessory			
Exercise name	**Equipment**	**Muscles used**	**Difficulty**
Lateral raise	DB	Mac	CBL	Delts	1
Tricep overhead extension	DB	CBL	Triceps	2
Tricep pushdown	CBL	Triceps	1
Close grip bench press	BB	Mac	Triceps	2
Bicep curl	DB	BB	CBL	Mac	Biceps	1
Hammer curl	DB	CBL	Mac	Biceps	1

Accessory exercises for 'lower' workout

Accessory			
Exercise name	**Equipment**	**Muscles used**	**Difficulty**
Seated leg curl	Mac	Hamstrings	1
Lying leg curl	Mac	Hamstrings	2
Leg extension	Mac	Quads	1
Standing calf raise	Mac	Calves	1
Bent knee calf raise	Mac	Calves	1

Additional Side Quest options for push-pull-legs splits

If doing a push-pull-legs split, you may choose to incorporate some additional 'Side Quest' exercises from the following options.

Accessory exercises for 'push' workout

Accessory			
Exercise name	**Equipment**	**Muscles used**	**Difficulty**
Lateral raise	DB | Mac | CBL	Delts	1
Tricep overhead extension	DB | CBL	Triceps	2
Tricep pushdown	CBL	Triceps	1
Close grip bench press	BB | Mac	Triceps	2
Tricep push-up	N/A	Triceps	2
Cable kick back	CBL	Triceps	1

Accessory exercises for 'pull' workout

Accessory			
Exercise name	**Equipment**	**Muscles used**	**Difficulty**
Lateral raise	DB | Mac | CBL	Delts	1
Face pull	CBL	Delts	1
Bicep curl	DB | BB | CBL	Biceps	1
Incline bicep curl	DB | CBL	Biceps	2
Preacher curl	DB | BB | Mac	Biceps	2
Hammer curl	DB | CBL	Biceps, Forearms	2
Reverse grip curl	DB | BB | CBL	Biceps, Forearms	2

Accessory exercises for 'legs' workout

Accessory			
Exercise name	**Equipment**	**Muscles used**	**Difficulty**
Seated leg curl	Mac	Hamstrings	1
Lying leg curl	Mac	Hamstrings	2
Leg extension	Mac	Quads	1
Standing calf raise	Mac	Calves	1
Bent knee calf raise	Mac	Calves	1

Which exercises use which muscles?

While you never need to learn complex exercise physiology, it can be helpful to learn which exercises train which parts of the body. And if you're trying to put together a split, such as push-pull-legs, this knowledge is essential. Here's a simple guide.

▶ **Squat** movements
will use these muscles:

Thighs (Quads)

Backs of thighs (Hamstrings)

Bum (Glutes)

▶ **Hinge** movements
will use these muscles:

Backs of thighs (Hamstrings)

Bum (Glutes)

Lower back (Erectors)

▶ **Lunge** movements
will use these muscles:

Thighs (Quads)

Backs of thighs (Hamstrings)

Bum (Glutes)

Calves

▶ **Pull** movements
will use these muscles:

Back (Lats)

Biceps

Forearms

Shoulders (Delts)

▶ **Push** movements
will use these muscles:

Chest (Pecs)

Shoulders (Delts)

Backs of arms (Triceps)

▶ **Core** movements
will use these muscles:

Abs (Abdominals)

Lower back (Erectors)

Sides of abs (Obliques)

▶ **Accessory** exercises:

Generally, the accessory exercises will target most of the muscles listed above. The difference is that they will typically be isolation movements, and they will involve fewer muscles compared to the compound movements.

Squat movements muscles

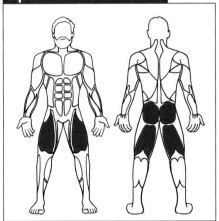

Pull movements muscles

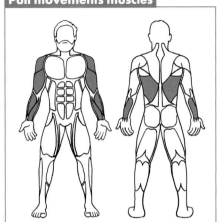

Hinge movements muscles

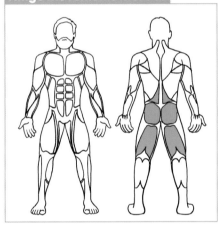

Push movements muscles

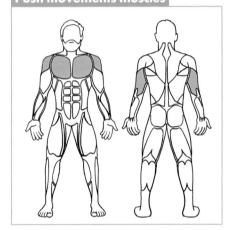

Lunge movements muscles

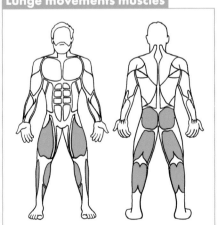

Core movements muscles

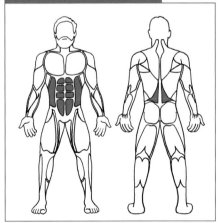

SAMPLE WORKOUTS

Depending on the type of workout you want to do, here are some ideas about how you might mix up the exercise options and put them together into a workout.

Sample full body workouts

Full body exercise list

	Squat
	Hinge
	Lunge
	Pull
	Push
	Core

Instructions: Do 8–12 reps of each of the exercises below.
Repeat for 2–3 sets.

Full body A

Movement	Exercise	Difficulty
Main Mission		
Squat	Goblet squat	1
Hinge	Hip thrust	1
Pull	Lat pulldown	1
Push	Incline bench press (DB)	2
Side Quest		
Core	Crunch	1
Lunge	Step-up	1

Full body B

Movement	Exercise	Difficulty
Main Mission		
Squat	Goblet squat	1
Hinge	Hip thrust	1
Lunge	Step-up	1
Pull	Lat pulldown	1
Side Quest		
Push	Incline bench press (DB)	2
Core	Crunch	1

Full body C

Movement	Exercise	Difficulty
Main Mission		
Hinge	Sumo deadlift	2
Lunge	Reverse lunge	3
Squat	Leg press	1
Pull	Seated row	1
Side Quest		
Push	Shoulder press	1
Core	Medicine ball slam	1

Sample upper-lower split workouts

Upper movement list

	Pull
	Push
	Core
	Accessory

Lower movement list

	Squat
	Hinge
	Lunge
	Core
	Accessory

Instructions: Do 8–12 reps of each of the exercises below. Repeat for 2–3 sets.

Hint: If you are making up your own workout rather than following this sample, select two pull exercises and two push exercises for your upper day; and one or more squat, hinge, and lunge on the lower day. Remember to note the level of difficulty when selecting your exercises. Also note that for this split, you have the additional option of including accessory work in your Side Quest.

Sample 'upper' workout

Movement		Exercise	Difficulty
Main Mission			
	Pull	Lat pulldown	1
	Push	Incline bench press	2
	Pull	Seated row	1
	Push	Shoulder press	1
Side Quest			
	Accessory	Tricep overhead extension	2
	Accessory	Bicep curl	1

Sample 'lower' workout

Movement		Exercise	Difficulty
Main Mission			
	Squat	Leg press	1
	Hinge	Trap bar deadlift	2
	Lunge	Step-up	1
	Hinge	Back extension	1
Side Quest			
	Accessory	Lying leg curl	1
	Core	Crunch	1

Sample push-pull-legs split workouts

Instructions: Do 8–12 reps of each of the exercises below. Repeat for 2–3 sets.

Hint: If you are making up your own workout rather than following this sample, select two or three pull exercises for your 'pull' day, and two or three push exercises for your 'push' day. Select at least one squat, hinge and lunge in your 'legs' day. Also note that for this split, you have the additional option of including accessory work.

Sample 'push' workout

Movement		Exercise	Difficulty
Main Mission			
	Push	Bench press	2
	Push	Assisted dip	1
	Push	Shoulder press	1
	Accessory	Crunch	1
Side Quest			
	Accessory	Tricep overhead extension	2
	Accessory	Tricep pushdown	1

Sample 'pull' workout

Movement		Exercise	Difficulty
Main Mission			
	Pull	Pull-up	3
	Pull	Seated row	1
	Pull	Lat pulldown	1
	Core	Deadbug	1
Side Quest			
	Accessory	Tricep overhead extension	2
	Accessory	Tricep pushdown	1

Sample 'legs' workout

Movement		Exercise	Difficulty
Main Mission			
	Squat	Back squat	3
	Hinge	Romanian deadlift	2
	Lunge	Static lunge	1
	Hinge	Back extension	1
Side Quest			
	Accessory	Leg extension	1
	Core	Medicine ball slam	1

SAMPLE SCHEDULES

To put everything into a weekly plan, here are some sample schedules to try. Remember, these are just ideas. You can organise your workouts into a schedule that works for you!

Weekly plan options for full body

Option a: alternating three workouts per week and two workouts per week (two-week split)

	Monday	Tuesday	Wednesday	Thursday	Friday	Saturday	Sunday
Week 1	Full body	Active recovery	Active recovery	Full body	Active recovery	Active recovery	Full body
Week 2	Active recovery	Full body	Active recovery	Active recovery	Full body	Active recovery	Active recovery

Option b: three workouts per week (two-week split)

	Monday	Tuesday	Wednesday	Thursday	Friday	Saturday	Sunday
Week 1	Full body	Active recovery	Full body	Active recovery	Full body	Active recovery	Active recovery
Week 2	Full body	Active recovery	Full body	Active recovery	Full body	Active recovery	Active recovery

Weekly plan options for upper-lower split

Option a: three workouts per week (two-week split)

	Monday	Tuesday	Wednesday	Thursday	Friday	Saturday	Sunday
Week 1	Upper	Active recovery	Lower	Active recovery	Upper	Active recovery	Active recovery
Week 2	Lower	Active recovery	Upper	Active recovery	Lower	Active recovery	Active recovery

Option b: four workouts per week (two-week split)

	Monday	Tuesday	Wednesday	Thursday	Friday	Saturday	Sunday
Week 1	Upper	Lower	Active recovery	Upper	Lower	Active recovery	Active recovery
Week 2	Upper	Lower	Active recovery	Upper	Lower	Active recovery	Active recovery

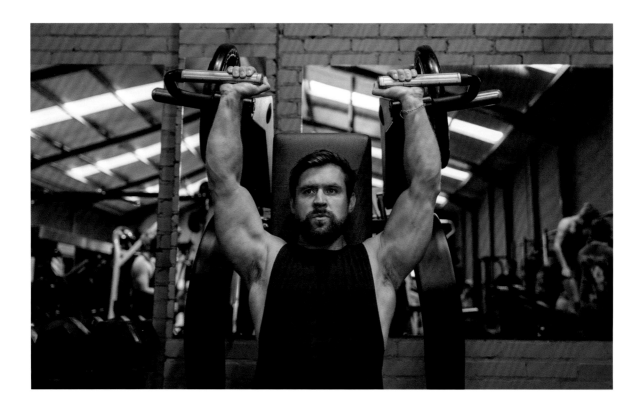

Weekly plan options for push-pull-legs

Option a: three workouts per week (two-week split)

	Monday	Tuesday	Wednesday	Thursday	Friday	Saturday	Sunday
Week 1	Push	Active recovery	Pull	Active recovery	Legs	Active recovery	Active recovery
Week 2	Push	Active recovery	Pull	Active recovery	Legs	Active recovery	Active recovery

Option b: four workouts per week (two-week split)

	Monday	Tuesday	Wednesday	Thursday	Friday	Saturday	Sunday
Week 1	Push	Legs	Active recovery	Pull	Legs	Active recovery	Active recovery
Week 2	Push	Legs	Active recovery	Pull	Legs	Active recovery	Active recovery

Option c: four workouts per week (three-week split)

	Monday	Tuesday	Wednesday	Thursday	Friday	Saturday	Sunday
Week 1	Push	Pull	Active recovery	Legs	Push	Active recovery	Active recovery
Week 2	Pull	Legs	Active recovery	Push	Pull	Active recovery	Active recovery
Week 3	Legs	Push	Active recovery	Pull	Legs	Active recovery	Active recovery

EXERCISE GUIDANCE

H ere's how to do each of the exercises referred to above.

Remember to maintain proper form throughout each exercise to prevent injury and maximise effectiveness. It's also important to choose weights that challenge you but still allow you to perform each exercise with control and proper technique.

For each exercise, repeat for the desired number of repetitions.

Squat

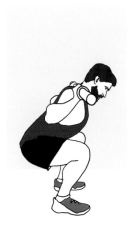

Barbell back squat

- Start by placing a barbell on a squat rack at about shoulder height.
- Step under the bar, positioning it across your upper back, resting it on your traps. Grip the bar wider than shoulder-width apart.
- Unrack the bar by straightening your legs, and step back to clear the rack.
- Stand with your feet shoulder-width apart or slightly wider, toes pointing slightly outwards.
- Brace your core and initiate the squat by pushing your hips back and bending your knees.

- Lower your body until your thighs are parallel to the ground or lower, keeping your chest up and back straight.
- Push through your heels to stand back up, extending your hips and knees.

Dumbbell goblet squat

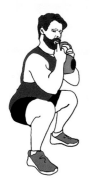

- Hold a dumbbell vertically against your chest with both hands, gripping the top of the dumbbell.
- Stand with your feet shoulder-width apart or slightly wider, toes pointing slightly outwards.
- Brace your core and squat down by pushing your hips back and bending your knees.
- Lower your body until your elbows touch the insides of your knees, keeping your chest up.
- Push through your heels to stand back up, extending your hips and knees.

Dumbbell suitcase squat

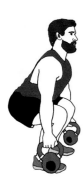

- Hold a dumbbell or kettlebell in each hand down by your side, like you're carrying suitcases.
- Stand with your feet shoulder-width apart or slightly wider, toes pointing forwards.
- Brace your core and squat down by pushing your hips back and bending your knees.
- Lower your body until your thighs are parallel to the ground or lower, keeping your chest up.
- Push through your heels to stand back up, extending your hips and knees.

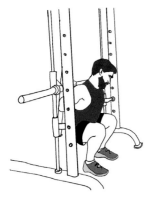

Smith machine squat

- Position yourself under the Smith machine bar with your feet shoulder-width apart or slightly wider.
- Rest the barbell across your upper back, with your hands slightly wider than shoulder-width apart.
- Brace your core and squat down by bending your knees and pushing your hips back.
- Lower your body until your thighs are parallel to the ground or lower, keeping your chest up.
- Push through your heels to stand back up, extending your hips and knees.

Machine hack squat

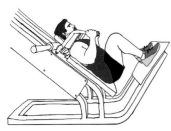

- Position yourself on the hack squat machine with your shoulders and back against the pads.
- Place your feet shoulder-width apart on the platform, with your toes pointing slightly outwards.
- Release the safety handles and brace your core.
- Lower the weight by bending your knees and hips until your thighs are parallel to the ground or lower.
- Push through your heels to extend your knees and hips, returning to the starting position.

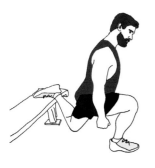

Dumbbell split squat

- Hold a dumbbell in each hand by your sides.
- Take a large step backwards with one foot and position it so that your back knee is bent.
- Keep your front foot flat on the ground, and your front knee bent at a 90-degree angle.
- Lower your body by bending both knees until your back knee is almost touching the ground.
- Push through your front heel to return to the starting position.

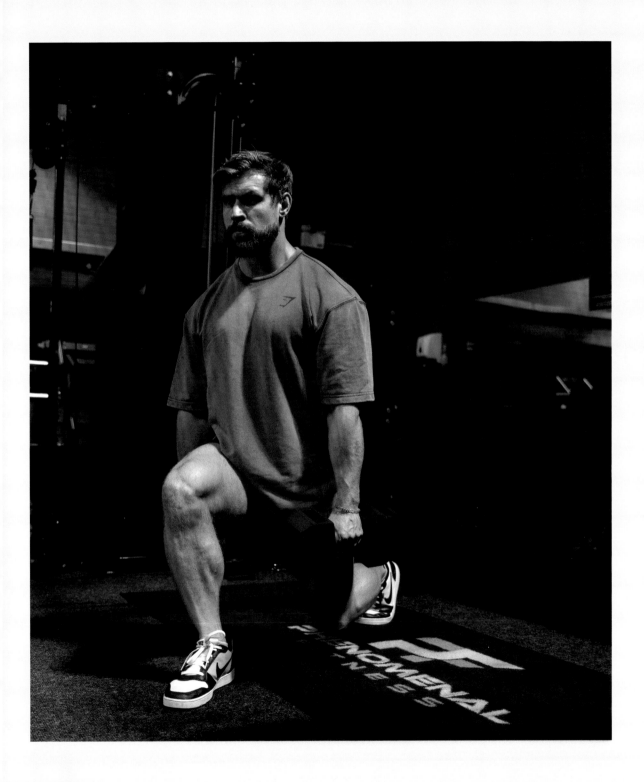

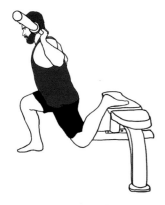

Barbell split squat

- Place a barbell across your upper back.
- Take a large step backwards with one foot and position it so that your back knee is bent and almost touching the ground.
- Keep your front foot flat on the ground, and your front knee bent at a 90-degree angle.
- Lower your body by bending both knees until your back knee is almost touching the ground.
- Push through your front heel to return to the starting position.

Machine leg press

- Sit on the leg-press machine with your back flat against the pad and your feet shoulder-width apart on the platform.
- Grip the handles on the sides of the seat for stability.
- Release the safety handles and brace your core.
- Lower the weight by bending your knees until they are at a 90-degree angle.
- Push through your heels to extend your knees and hips, returning to the starting position.

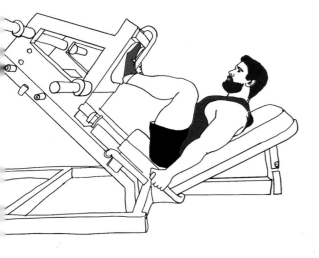

Hinge

Barbell deadlift

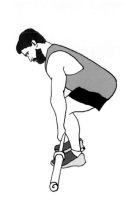

- Stand with your feet about hip-width apart, toes pointing forwards, and a barbell on the floor in front of you.
- Bend at your hips and knees to lower yourself down and grasp the bar with an overhand grip, hands slightly wider than shoulder-width apart.
- Keep your back straight, chest up and core engaged.
- Drive through your heels, extending your hips and knees simultaneously to lift the barbell off the ground.
- As you stand up, keep the bar close to your body and straighten your back.
- Once you're standing fully upright, slowly lower the bar back down by reversing the movement.
- Keep the bar close to your body throughout the entire lift to maintain proper form and prevent injury.

Trap bar deadlift

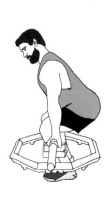

- Stand inside a trap bar (hex bar) with your feet about hip-width apart.
- Bend at your hips and knees to grasp the handles of the trap bar, keeping your back straight, chest up and core engaged.
- Drive through your heels, extending your hips and knees simultaneously to lift the trap bar off the ground.
- As you stand up, keep your back straight and chest up.
- Once you're standing fully upright, slowly lower the trap bar back down by reversing the movement.
- Maintain proper form throughout the lift, keeping the trap bar close to your body.

Barbell sumo deadlift

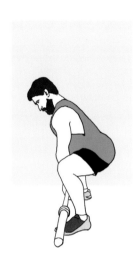

- Stand with your feet wider than shoulder-width apart and your toes pointed outwards at about a 45-degree angle.
- Position a barbell in front of you with your hands gripping the barbell between your legs, using a wider grip than a conventional deadlift.
- Bend at your hips and knees to grasp the barbell with an overhand grip, keeping your back straight, chest up and core engaged.
- Drive through your heels and extend your hips and knees simultaneously to lift the barbell off the ground.
- As you stand up, keep your back straight and chest up.
- Once you're standing fully upright, slowly lower the barbell back down by reversing the movement.
- Maintain proper form throughout the lift, focusing on keeping your back straight and chest up.

Machine back extension

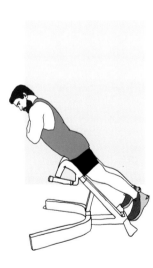

- Adjust the back-extension machine so that the pad is positioned at the top of your thighs.
- Stand on the platform with your feet shoulder-width apart and your toes pointed forwards.
- Cross your arms over your chest or place your hands behind your head.
- Lower your upper body towards the ground by bending at your hips, keeping your back straight.
- Once you reach a comfortable stretch in your hamstrings, reverse the movement by extending your hips and returning to the starting position.
- Squeeze your glutes at the top of the movement to engage your lower back muscles.
- Avoid hyperextending your lower back at the top of the movement.

Barbell hip thrust

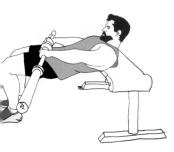

- Sit on the ground with your upper back against a bench and a barbell across your hips.
- Roll the barbell over your hips so that it's directly above your pelvis.
- Bend your knees and place your feet flat on the ground, hip-width apart.
- Brace your core and drive through your heels to lift your hips towards the ceiling until your body forms a straight line from your shoulders to your knees.
- Squeeze your glutes at the top of the movement, then lower your hips back down under control.

Machine hip thrust

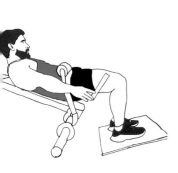

- Sit on the machine with your upper back against the padded support and your feet flat on the footplate.
- Adjust the seat height and footplate position so that your knees are at about a 90-degree angle when your hips are fully extended.
- Place a pad or barbell across your hips for added resistance.
- Brace your core and drive through your heels to extend your hips and lift the weight until your body forms a straight line.
- Squeeze your glutes at the top of the movement, then lower the weight back down under control.

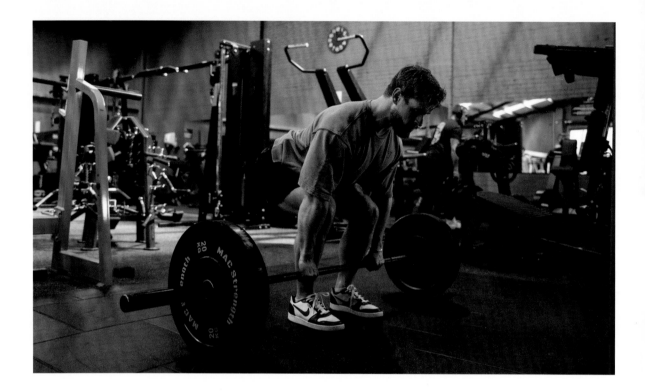

Barbell Romanian deadlift

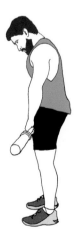

- Stand with your feet about hip-width apart, toes pointed forwards, and hold a barbell in front of your thighs with an overhand grip, hands slightly wider than shoulder-width apart.
- Brace your core, keep your back straight and slightly bend your knees.
- Hinge at your hips, pushing your hips back as you lower the barbell towards the ground while maintaining a slight bend in your knees.
- Lower the barbell until you feel a stretch in your hamstrings or until your back starts to curve but keep the bar close to your body.
- Keep your back straight throughout the movement and avoid curving your spine.
- Drive through your heels and squeeze your glutes to return to the starting position.

Lunge

Dumbbell static lunge

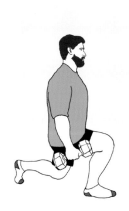

- Hold a dumbbell in each hand, with your arms at your sides.
- Take a step forward with one foot and a step back with the other foot, creating a staggered stance.
- Lower your body by bending both knees until your back knee is just above the ground and your front thigh is parallel to the ground.
- Keep your torso upright and your chest up throughout the movement.
- Push through the heel of your front foot to return to the starting position.
- Repeat for the desired number of repetitions, then switch legs and repeat.

Barbell static lunge

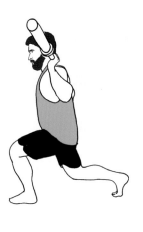

- Place a barbell across your upper back.
- Take a step forward with one foot and a step back with the other foot, creating a staggered stance.
- Lower your body by bending both knees until your back knee is just above the ground and your front thigh is parallel to the ground.
- Keep your torso upright and your chest up throughout the movement.
- Push through the heel of your front foot to return to the starting position.
- Repeat for the desired number of repetitions, then switch legs and repeat.

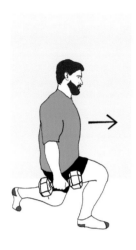

Dumbbell walking lunge

- Hold a dumbbell in each hand, with your arms at your sides.
- Take a step forward with one foot and lower your body by bending both knees until your back knee is just above the ground and your front thigh is parallel to the ground.
- Push through the heel of your front foot to step forwards and bring your back foot forwards to meet the front foot.
- Repeat the movement, alternating legs with each step.
- Continue walking forwards for the desired distance or number of repetitions.

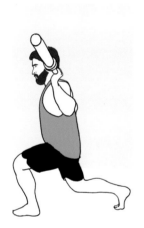

Barbell walking lunge

- Place a barbell across your upper back.
- Take a step forward with one foot and lower your body by bending both knees until your back knee is just above the ground and your front thigh is parallel to the ground.
- Push through the heel of your front foot to step forwards and bring your back foot forwards to meet the front foot.
- Repeat the movement, alternating legs with each step.
- Continue walking forwards for the desired distance or number of repetitions.

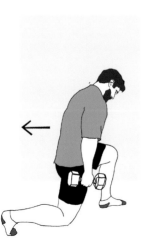

Dumbbell reverse lunge

- Hold a dumbbell in each hand, with your arms at your sides.
- Take a step backwards with one foot and lower your body by bending both knees until your back knee is just above the ground and your front thigh is parallel to the ground.
- Keep your torso upright and your chest up throughout the movement.
- Push through the heel of your front foot to return to the starting position.
- Repeat for the desired number of repetitions, then switch legs and repeat.

Barbell reverse lunge

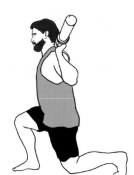

- Place a barbell across your upper back.
- Take a step backwards with one foot and lower your body by bending both knees until your back knee is just above the ground and your front thigh is parallel to the ground.
- Keep your torso upright and your chest up throughout the movement.
- Push through the heel of your front foot to return to the starting position.
- Repeat for the desired number of repetitions, then switch legs and repeat.

Dumbbell front elevated lunge

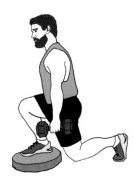

- Hold a dumbbell in each hand, with your arms at your sides.
- Place one foot on a raised platform, such as a bench or step, and step back with the other foot.
- Lower your body by bending both knees until your back knee is just above the ground and your front thigh is parallel to the ground.
- Keep your torso upright and your chest up throughout the movement.
- Push through the heel of your front foot to return to the starting position.
- Repeat for the desired number of repetitions, then switch legs and repeat.

Barbell front elevated lunge

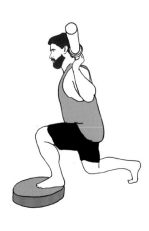

- Place a barbell across your upper back.
- Place one foot on a raised platform, such as a bench or step, and step backwards with the other foot.
- Lower your body by bending both knees until your back knee is just above the ground and your front thigh is parallel to the ground.
- Keep your torso upright and your chest up throughout the movement.
- Push through the heel of your front foot to return to the starting position.
- Repeat for the desired number of repetitions, then switch legs and repeat.

Dumbbell lateral lunge

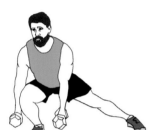

- Hold a dumbbell in each hand, with your arms at your sides.
- Take a step to the side with one foot, keeping the other foot planted.
- Lower your body by bending the knee of the stepping leg, while keeping the other leg straight.
- Keep your torso upright and your chest up throughout the movement.
- Push through the heel of the stepping leg to return to the starting position.
- Repeat for the desired number of repetitions, then switch legs and repeat.

Barbell lateral lunge

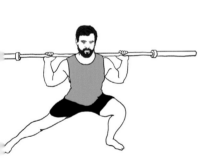

- Place a barbell across your upper back.
- Take a step to the side with one foot, keeping the other foot planted.
- Lower your body by bending the knee of the stepping leg, while keeping the other leg straight.
- Keep your torso upright and your chest up throughout the movement.
- Push through the heel of the stepping leg to return to the starting position.
- Repeat for the desired number of repetitions, then switch legs and repeat.

Dumbbell step-up

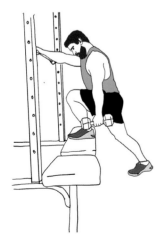

- Hold a dumbbell in each hand, with your arms at your sides.
- Stand facing a sturdy bench or platform.
- Place one foot flat on the bench or platform and push through the heel of that foot to step up onto the bench.
- Keep your chest up and your back straight throughout the movement.
- Step back down with control, returning to the starting position.
- Repeat for the desired number of repetitions on one leg before switching to the other leg.

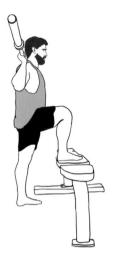

Barbell step-up

- Place a barbell across your upper back.
- Stand facing a sturdy bench or platform.
- Place one foot flat on the bench or platform and push through the heel of that foot to step up onto the bench.
- Keep your chest up and your back straight throughout the movement.
- Step back down with control, returning to the starting position.
- Repeat for the desired number of repetitions on one leg before switching to the other leg.

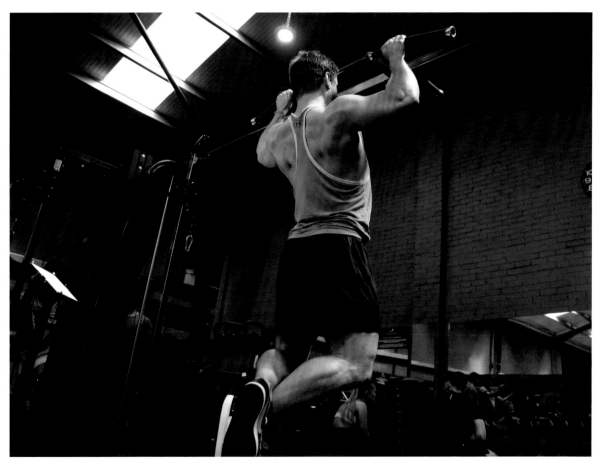

Pull

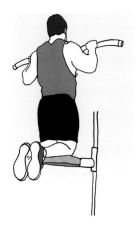

Machine assisted pull-up

- Adjust the machine's weight stack to an appropriate resistance.
- Step onto the foot platform and grip the handles or bar with an overhand grip.
- Hang from the handles with your arms fully extended and your shoulders relaxed.
- Pull yourself up by bending your elbows and pulling your chest towards the handles.
- Keep your chest up and your shoulders pulled back throughout the movement.
- Lower yourself back down with control until your arms are fully extended.

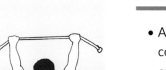

Machine lat pulldown

- Adjust the thigh pads and seat height of the machine to fit your body comfortably.
- Sit down and grip the bar with your hands slightly wider than shoulder-width apart, palms facing forwards.
- Brace your core and pull the bar down towards your chest by bending your elbows and squeezing your shoulder blades together.
- Keep your chest up and your back straight throughout the movement.
- Slowly return the bar to the starting position, fully extending your arms.

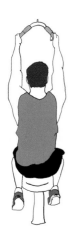

Machine neutral grip pulldown

- Adjust the thigh pads and seat height of the machine to fit your body comfortably.
- Sit down and grip the bar with your hands using a neutral grip (palms facing each other) on the handles.
- Perform the pulldown motion by bending your elbows and pulling the handles towards your chest.
- Keep your chest up and your back straight throughout the movement.
- Slowly return the handles to the starting position, fully extending your arms.

Cable neutral grip pulldown

- Attach a long bar or D-handle to the cable pulley machine at the highest position.
- Grip the handle with both hands using a neutral grip (palms facing each other).
- Step back a few feet from the machine and kneel down on one knee or stand with a staggered stance for stability.
- Pull the handle down towards your chest by bending your elbows and squeezing your shoulder blades together.
- Keep your chest up and your back straight throughout the movement.
- Slowly return the handle to the starting position, fully extending your arms.

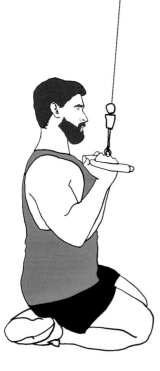

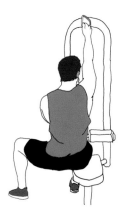

Machine one-arm pulldown

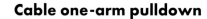

- Adjust the weight stack and seat height of the machine as needed.
- Sit down and grip the handle with one hand, palm facing forwards.
- Brace your core and pull the handle down towards your chest by bending your elbow and squeezing your shoulder blade.
- Keep your chest up and your back straight throughout the movement.
- Slowly return the handle to the starting position, fully extending your arm.
- Repeat for the desired number of repetitions on one side before switching to the other side.

Cable one-arm pulldown

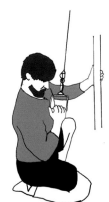

- Attach a single handle to the cable pulley machine at the highest position.
- Grip the handle with one hand, palm facing forwards.
- Step back a few feet from the machine and kneel on one knee or stand with a staggered stance for stability.
- Pull the handle down towards your chest by bending your elbow and squeezing your shoulder blade.
- Keep your chest up and your back straight throughout the movement.
- Slowly return the handle to the starting position, fully extending your arm.
- Repeat for the desired number of repetitions on one side before switching to the other side.

Cable machine supinated pulldown

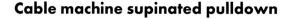

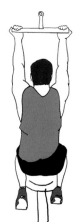

- Sit down and grip the bar with your hands using an underhand grip (palms facing you) on the handles.
- Perform the pulldown motion by bending your elbows and pulling the bar down towards your chest.
- Keep your chest up and your back straight throughout the movement.
- Slowly return the bar to the starting position, fully extending your arms.

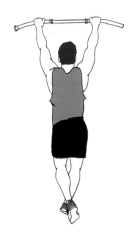

Pull-up

- Grip a pull-up bar with your hands slightly wider than shoulder-width apart, palms facing away from you (overhand grip).
- Hang from the bar with your arms fully extended and your shoulders relaxed.
- Pull yourself up by bending your elbows and pulling your chin above the bar.
- Keep your chest up and your shoulders pulled back throughout the movement.
- Lower yourself back down with control until your arms are fully extended.

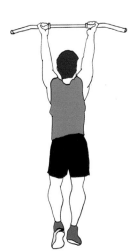

Chin-up

- Grip a pull-up bar with your hands shoulder-width apart or slightly narrower, palms facing towards you (underhand grip).
- Hang from the bar with your arms fully extended and your shoulders relaxed.
- Pull yourself up by bending your elbows and pulling your chin above the bar.
- Keep your chest up and your shoulders pulled back throughout the movement.
- Lower yourself back down with control until your arms are fully extended.

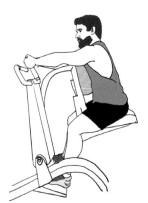

Machine seated row

- Adjust the seat and footplate of the machine to fit your body comfortably.
- Sit down and grip the handles with an overhand grip, palms facing down.
- Brace your core and pull the handles towards your lower chest by retracting your shoulder blades and squeezing your back muscles.
- Keep your chest up and your back straight throughout the movement.
- Slowly return the handles to the starting position, fully extending your arms.

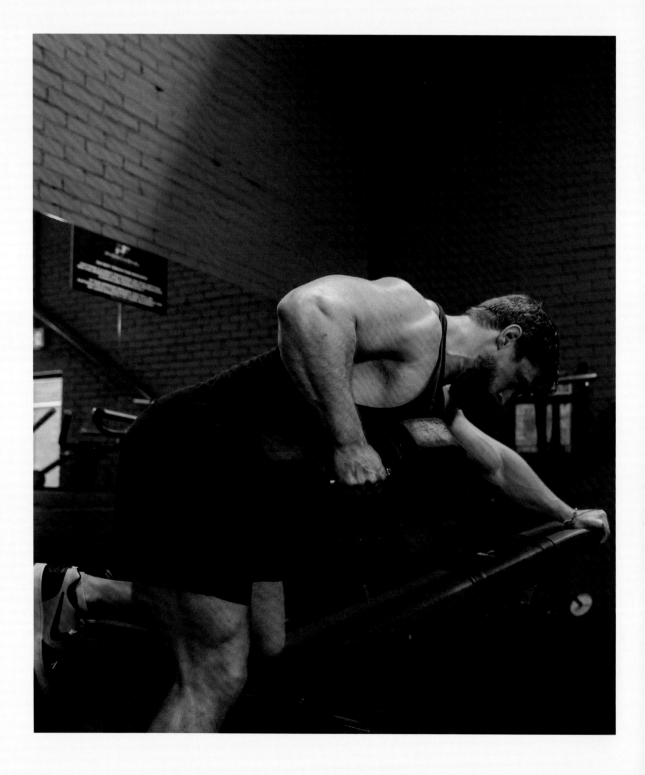

Cable seated row

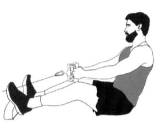

- Sit down on a bench or seat facing the cable pulley machine with your feet stablised on the foot plates and knees slightly bent.
- Grip the handle with a neutral grip, palms facing towards each other.
- Brace your core and pull the handle towards your lower chest by retracting your shoulder blades and squeezing your back muscles.
- Keep your chest up and your back straight throughout the movement.
- Slowly return the handle to the starting position, fully extending your arms.

Dumbbell seated row

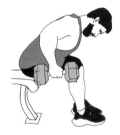

- Sit down on a bench or seat with a dumbbell in each hand, palms facing each other.
- Lean forward slightly with your chest up and your back straight.
- Pull the dumbbells towards your lower chest by retracting your shoulder blades and squeezing your back muscles.
- Keep your chest up and your back straight throughout the movement.
- Slowly lower the dumbbells back down to the starting position, fully extending your arms.

Machine single-arm row

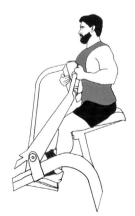

- Adjust the seat and footplate of the machine to fit your body comfortably.
- Sit down and grip the handle with one hand, palm facing down.
- Brace your core and pull the handle towards your lower chest by retracting your shoulder blade and squeezing your back muscles.
- Keep your chest up and your back straight throughout the movement.
- Slowly return the handle to the starting position, fully extending your arm.
- Repeat for the desired number of repetitions on one side before switching to the other side.

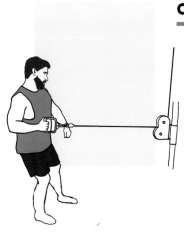

Cable single-arm row

- Attach a single handle to the cable pulley machine at about waist height.
- Stand facing the machine with one foot forward and one foot back, knees slightly bent.
- Grip the handle with one hand, palm facing down.
- Brace your core and pull the handle towards your lower chest by retracting your shoulder blade and squeezing your back muscles.
- Keep your chest up and your back straight throughout the movement.
- Slowly return the handle to the starting position, fully extending your arm.
- Repeat for the desired number of repetitions on one side before switching to the other side.

Dumbbell single-arm row

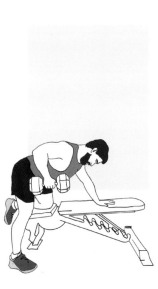

- Stand with your feet shoulder-width apart, holding a dumbbell in one hand.
- Hinge at your hips and bend your knees slightly, keeping your back straight and chest up.
- Let the dumbbell hang down towards the floor.
- Pull the dumbbell up towards your hip by retracting your shoulder blade and squeezing your back muscles.
- Keep your chest up and your back straight throughout the movement.
- Slowly lower the dumbbell back down to the starting position, fully extending your arm.
- Repeat for the desired number of repetitions on one side before switching to the other side.

Cable bent-over row

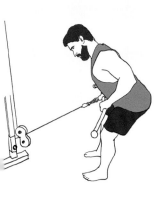

- Attach a straight or angled bar to the cable pulley machine at about waist height.
- Stand facing the machine with your feet shoulder-width apart and knees slightly bent.
- Grip the bar with an overhand grip, hands slightly wider than shoulder-width apart.
- Hinge at your hips and bend forwards at about a 45-degree angle, keeping your back straight and chest up.
- Pull the bar towards your lower chest by retracting your shoulder blades and squeezing your back muscles.
- Keep your chest up and your back straight throughout the movement.
- Slowly return the bar to the starting position, fully extending your arms.

Barbell bent-over row

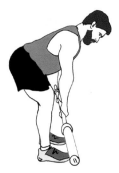

- Stand with your feet shoulder-width apart, holding a barbell with a shoulder width grip.
- Hinge at your hips and bend forwards at about a 45-degree angle, keeping your back straight and chest up.
- Let the barbell hang down towards the floor.
- Pull the barbell up towards your lower chest by retracting your shoulder blades and squeezing your back muscles.
- Keep your chest up and your back straight throughout the movement.
- Slowly lower the barbell back down to the starting position, fully extending your arms.

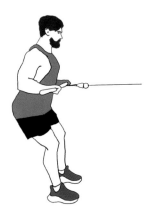

Cable supinated row

- Attach a straight or angled bar to the cable pulley machine at about waist height.
- Stand facing the machine with your feet shoulder-width apart and knees slightly bent.
- Grip the bar with an underhand grip (palms facing up), hands slightly wider than shoulder-width apart.
- Pull the bar towards your lower chest by retracting your shoulder blades and squeezing your back muscles.
- Keep your chest up and your back straight throughout the movement.
- Slowly return the bar to the starting position, fully extending your arms.

Dumbbell supinated row

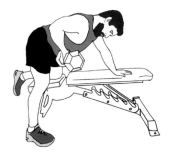

- Stand with your feet shoulder-width apart, holding a dumbbell in each hand.
- Hinge at your hips and bend forwards at about a 45-degree angle, keeping your back straight and chest up.
- Grip the dumbbells with an underhand grip (palms facing up), hands slightly wider than shoulder-width apart.
- Pull the dumbbells up towards your lower chest by retracting your shoulder blades and squeezing your back muscles.
- Keep your chest up and your back straight throughout the movement.
- Slowly lower the dumbbells back down to the starting position, fully extending your arms.

Barbell inverted row

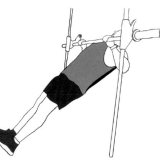

- Set up a barbell in a power rack or Smith machine at about waist height.
- Lie on your back underneath the barbell with your arms fully extended, gripping the barbell with an overhand grip, hands slightly wider than shoulder-width apart.
- Keep your body in a straight line from your head to your heels.
- Brace your core and pull your chest towards the barbell by bending your elbows and squeezing your shoulder blades together.
- Keep your body in a straight line throughout the movement.
- Slowly lower yourself back down to the starting position, fully extending your arms.

Machine T-bar row

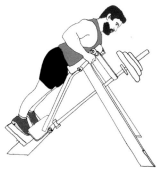

- Position yourself in front of the T-bar row machine with your feet shoulder-width apart and knees slightly bent.
- Straddle the barbell and grip the handles or the V-bar attachment with an overhand grip.
- Brace your core and pull the handles or the V-bar towards your lower chest by retracting your shoulder blades and squeezing your back muscles.
- Keep your chest up and your back straight throughout the movement.
- Slowly return the handles or the V-bar to the starting position, fully extending your arms.

Push

Dumbbell bench press

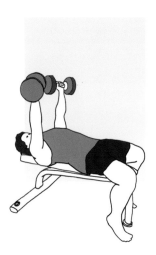

- Lie flat on a bench with a dumbbell in each hand, palms facing away from you.
- Hold the dumbbells above your chest with your arms fully extended.
- Lower the dumbbells down towards your chest while keeping your elbows slightly bent.
- Pause when your elbows are just below the level of the bench.
- Push the dumbbells back up to the starting position, fully extending your arms.

Barbell bench press

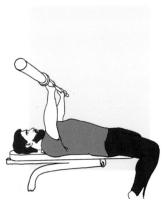

- Lie flat on a bench with your feet firmly planted on the ground.
- Grip the barbell with your hands slightly wider than shoulder-width apart, palms facing away from you.
- Unrack the barbell and hold it above your chest with your arms fully extended.
- Lower the barbell down towards your chest, keeping your elbows slightly tucked.
- Touch the barbell to your chest or just above it.
- Push the barbell back up to the starting position, fully extending your arms.

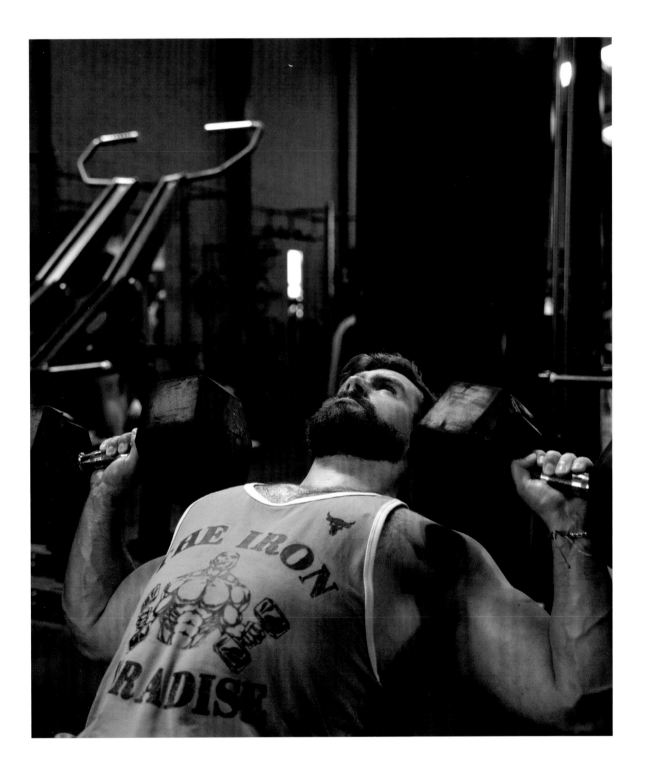

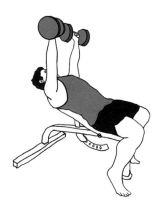

Dumbbell incline bench press

- Adjust a bench to a 30–45 degree incline.
- Lie back on the bench with a dumbbell in each hand, palms facing away from you.
- Hold the dumbbells above your chest with your arms fully extended.
- Lower the dumbbells down towards your chest while keeping your elbows slightly bent.
- Push the dumbbells back up to the starting position, fully extending your arms.

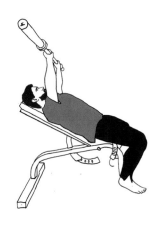

Barbell incline bench press

- Adjust a bench to a 30–45 degree incline.
- Lie back on the bench with your feet firmly planted on the ground.
- Grip the barbell with your hands slightly wider than shoulder-width apart, palms facing away from you.
- Unrack the barbell and hold it above your chest with your arms fully extended.
- Lower the barbell down towards your chest, keeping your elbows slightly tucked.
- Push the barbell back up to the starting position, fully extending your arms.

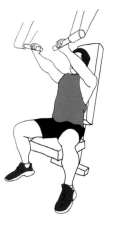

Machine incline bench press

- Adjust the seat and backrest of the machine to a 30–45 degree incline.
- Sit down on the machine and grip the handles with your palms facing away from you.
- Push the handles away from your body to extend your arms fully.
- Lower the handles down towards your chest, keeping your elbows slightly bent.
- Push the handles back up to the starting position, fully extending your arms.

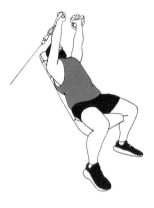

Cable incline bench press

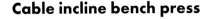

- Adjust a bench to a 30–45 degree incline and position it in front of a cable machine.
- Attach handles to the high pulleys of the cable machine.
- Sit down on the bench and grip the handles with your palms facing away from you.
- Push the handles away from your body to extend your arms fully.
- Lower the handles down towards your chest, keeping your elbows slightly bent.
- Push the handles back up to the starting position, fully extending your arms.

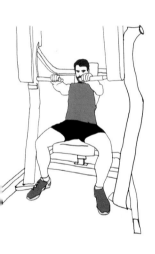

Machine chest press

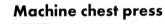

- Adjust the seat and handles of the machine to fit your body comfortably.
- Sit down on the machine and grip the handles with your palms facing away from you.
- Push the handles away from your body to extend your arms fully.
- Lower the handles towards your chest, keeping your elbows slightly bent.
- Push the handles back up to the starting position, fully extending your arms.

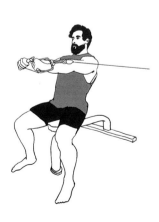

Cable chest press

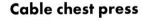

- Attach handles to the high pulleys of a cable machine.
- Stand facing away from the machine with one foot in front of the other for stability.
- Grip the handles with your palms facing away from you.
- Push the handles away from your body to extend your arms fully.
- Bring the handles towards your chest, keeping your elbows slightly bent.
- Push the handles back out to the starting position, fully extending your arms.

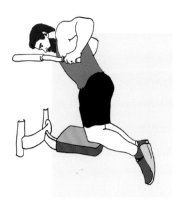

Machine assisted dips

- Adjust the machine to an appropriate weight.
- Step onto the foot platform and grip the handles with your palms facing inwards.
- Lower your body by bending your elbows until your upper arms are parallel to the ground.
- Push through your palms to extend your elbows and return to the starting position.

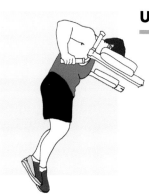

Unassisted dips

- Grip parallel bars with your palms facing inwards.
- Lift yourself up so your arms are fully extended and your feet are off the ground.
- Lower your body by bending your elbows until your upper arms are parallel to the ground.
- Push through your palms to extend your elbows and return to the starting position.

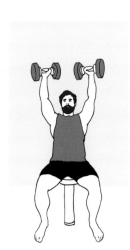

Dumbbell shoulder press

- Sit on a bench with a dumbbell in each hand, palms facing forwards.
- Hold the dumbbells at shoulder height with your elbows bent and pointing out to the sides.
- Press the dumbbells overhead until your arms are fully extended.
- Lower the dumbbells back down to shoulder height with control.

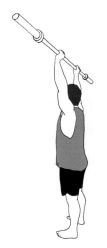

Barbell shoulder press

- Sit on a bench with a barbell racked at shoulder height.
- Grip the barbell with your hands slightly wider than shoulder-width apart, palms facing forwards.
- Unrack the barbell and hold it at shoulder height with your elbows bent and pointing out to the sides.
- Press the barbell overhead until your arms are fully extended.
- Lower the barbell back down to shoulder height with control.

Machine shoulder press

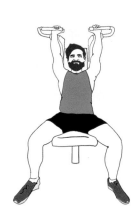

- Adjust the seat and handles of the machine to fit your body comfortably.
- Sit down on the machine and grip the handles with your palms facing forwards.
- Press the handles overhead until your arms are fully extended.
- Lower the handles back down to shoulder height with control.

Dumbbell single-arm shoulder press

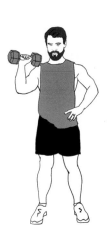

- Sit on a bench with a dumbbell in one hand, palm facing forwards.
- Hold the dumbbell at shoulder height with your elbow bent and pointing out to the side.
- Press the dumbbell overhead until your arm is fully extended.
- Lower the dumbbell back down to shoulder height with control.
- Repeat for the desired number of repetitions on one side before switching to the other side.

Core

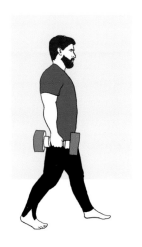

Dumbbell suitcase carry

- Stand upright with a dumbbell in one hand and your arm fully extended by your side.
- Keep your shoulder blades pulled back and down, and your chest up.
- Engage your core muscles to stabilise your torso.
- Begin walking forwards while maintaining an upright posture and keeping the dumbbell at your side.
- Walk for a predetermined distance or time, ensuring that you keep your torso stable and avoid leaning to one side.
- Switch the dumbbell to the opposite hand and repeat the walk.

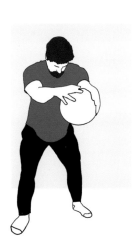

Medicine ball slam

- Stand with your feet shoulder-width apart, holding a medicine ball overhead with both hands.
- Engage your core muscles and maintain a straight back.
- Explosively slam the medicine ball down to the ground in front of you as hard as you can.
- As you slam the ball, bend your knees and hinge at your hips to generate power from your lower body.
- Catch the ball on the rebound or let it hit the ground and squat down to pick it up, then immediately repeat the movement for the desired number of repetitions.

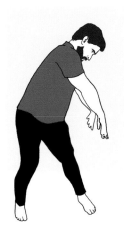

Medicine ball side slam

- Stand sideways to a wall or an open space with your feet shoulder-width apart.
- Hold a medicine ball with both hands at one side of your body, keeping your arms extended.
- Engage your core muscles and maintain a straight back.
- Explosively slam the medicine ball down to the ground on the side of your body, rotating your torso and bending your knees slightly.
- As you slam the ball, use your oblique muscles to generate power and rotate your torso.
- Catch the ball on the rebound or let it hit the ground and squat down to pick it up, then immediately repeat the movement on the opposite side for the desired number of repetitions.

Bicycle crunch

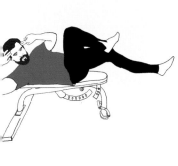

- Lie on your back on the floor with your hands behind your head, elbows pointing out to the sides.
- Lift your legs off the ground and bend your knees to a 90-degree angle.
- Engage your core muscles to lift your shoulder blades off the ground.
- Simultaneously rotate your torso and bring your right elbow towards your left knee while straightening your right leg.
- At the same time, extend your left leg out straight, hovering above the ground.
- Alternate sides, bringing your left elbow towards your right knee while straightening your left leg.
- Continue alternating sides in a pedalling motion, keeping your core engaged throughout the exercise.

Deadbug

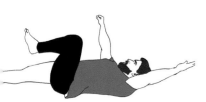

- Lie on your back on the floor with your arms extended towards the ceiling and your legs bent at a 90-degree angle.
- Engage your core muscles to press your lower back into the floor.
- Slowly lower your right arm and left leg towards the ground, maintaining a stable core and keeping your lower back pressed into the floor.
- Return to the starting position and repeat with the opposite arm and leg.
- Continue alternating sides in a controlled manner, focusing on maintaining stability and avoiding arching your lower back.

Bird dog

- Start on your hands and knees in a tabletop position, with your wrists aligned under your shoulders and your knees under your hips.
- Engage your core muscles to stabilise your spine.
- Extend your right arm straight out in front of you while simultaneously extending your left leg straight back behind you.
- Keep your hips and shoulders squared to the ground, avoiding any rotation or tilting.
- Hold this position briefly, then return to the starting position.
- Repeat with the opposite arm and leg, extending your left arm and right leg.
- Continue alternating sides while maintaining stability and control throughout the movement.

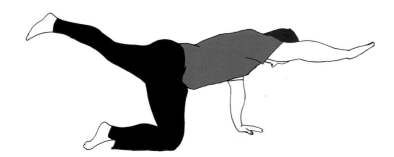

Crunch

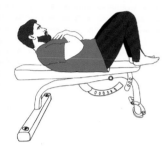

- Lie on your back on the floor with your knees bent and feet flat on the ground, hip-width apart.
- Place your hands behind your head or cross them over your chest.
- Engage your core muscles to lift your shoulder blades off the ground, curling your upper body towards your knees.
- Keep your lower back pressed into the floor and avoid pulling on your neck with your hands.
- Exhale as you crunch up, and inhale as you lower back down to the starting position.
- Repeat for the desired number of repetitions, focusing on controlled movements and maintaining tension in your abdominal muscles throughout the exercise.

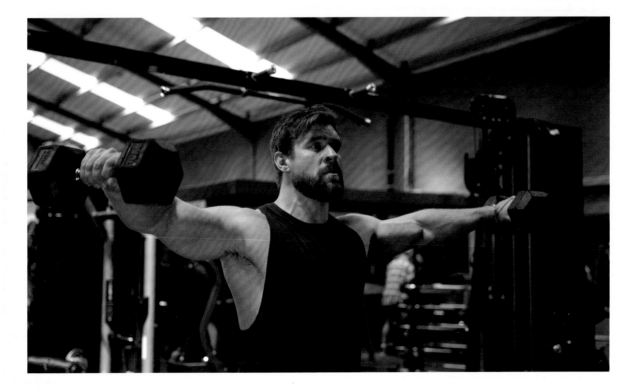

Accessory (upper body)

Dumbbell lateral raises

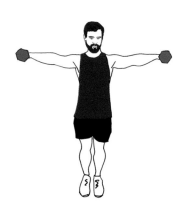

- Stand upright with a dumbbell in each hand, palms facing towards your body.
- Keep a slight bend in your elbows and maintain a neutral spine.
- Engage your core muscles for stability.
- Raise the dumbbells out to the sides until your arms are parallel to the ground, or slightly below shoulder level.
- Keep your wrists straight throughout the movement.
- Slowly lower the dumbbells back down to the starting position.

Machine lateral raises

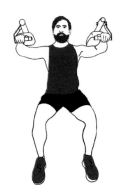

- Adjust the seat height and handles of the lateral raise machine so that your arms are in line with the machine's pivot point.
- Sit down on the machine with your back against the pad and grip the handles.
- Keep your chest up, shoulders back, and core engaged.
- Raise the handles out to the sides until your arms are parallel to the ground.
- Slowly lower the handles back down to the starting position.

Cable lateral raises

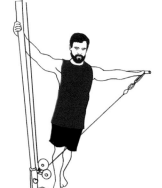

- Stand facing a cable machine with the handle attached to the low pulley.
- Hold the handle with one hand and step away from the machine to create tension in the cable.
- Keep a slight bend in your elbow and your palm facing downwards.
- Raise the handle out to the side until your arm is parallel to the ground.
- Slowly lower the handle back down to the starting position.
- Repeat for the desired number of repetitions on one side before switching to the other side.

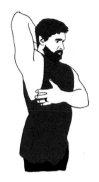

Dumbbell tricep overhead extension

- Stand or sit on a bench with a dumbbell in one hand.
- Hold the dumbbell with both hands and raise it overhead, keeping your elbows close to your ears and your palms facing upwards.
- Lower the dumbbell behind your head by bending your elbows, allowing them to hinge only at the elbow joint.
- Keep your upper arms stationary and your core engaged.
- Extend your arms to raise the dumbbell back to the starting position.

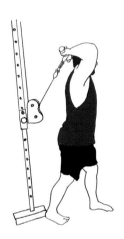

Cable tricep overhead extension

- Attach a rope handle to a high pulley on a cable machine.
- Stand facing away from the machine and grip the handle with both hands.
- Step forwards slightly and lean forwards, keeping your back straight.
- Extend your arms overhead, keeping your elbows close to your ears and your palms facing each other.
- Lower the rope behind your head by bending your elbows, allowing them to hinge only at the elbow joint.
- Keep your upper arms stationary and your core engaged.
- Extend your arms to raise the rope back to the starting position.

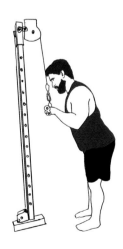

Cable tricep pushdown

- Attach a straight or angled bar to a high pulley on a cable machine.
- Stand facing the machine and grip the bar with both hands, palms facing down.
- Keep your elbows close to your sides and your upper arms stationary.
- Push the bar downwards by straightening your elbows, focusing on contracting your triceps.
- Keep your core engaged and avoid leaning forwards or using momentum.
- Slowly return the bar to the starting position by bending your elbows.

Barbell close grip bench press

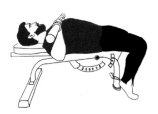

- Lie flat on a bench with your feet flat on the ground and grip the barbell with your hands closer than shoulder-width apart, palms facing away from you.
- Unrack the barbell and hold it directly above your chest with your arms fully extended.
- Lower the barbell towards your chest while keeping your elbows close to your sides.
- Pause briefly when the barbell touches your chest, then press it back up to the starting position, fully extending your arms.

Machine close grip bench press

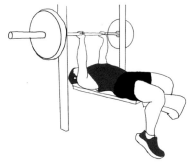

- Adjust the seat and handles of the machine to fit your body comfortably.
- Sit down on the machine and grip the handles with your hands closer than shoulder-width apart.
- Press the handles forwards until your arms are fully extended.
- Bring the handles towards your chest while keeping your elbows close to your sides.
- Pause briefly when the handles are close to your chest, then press them back up to the starting position, fully extending your arms.

Dumbbell bicep curls

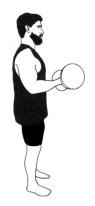

- Stand upright with a dumbbell in each hand, arms fully extended by your sides, palms facing forwards.
- Keep your elbows close to your sides and your core engaged.
- Curl the dumbbells upwards towards your shoulders by bending your elbows, keeping your upper arms stationary.
- Squeeze your biceps at the top of the movement.
- Slowly lower the dumbbells back down to the starting position.

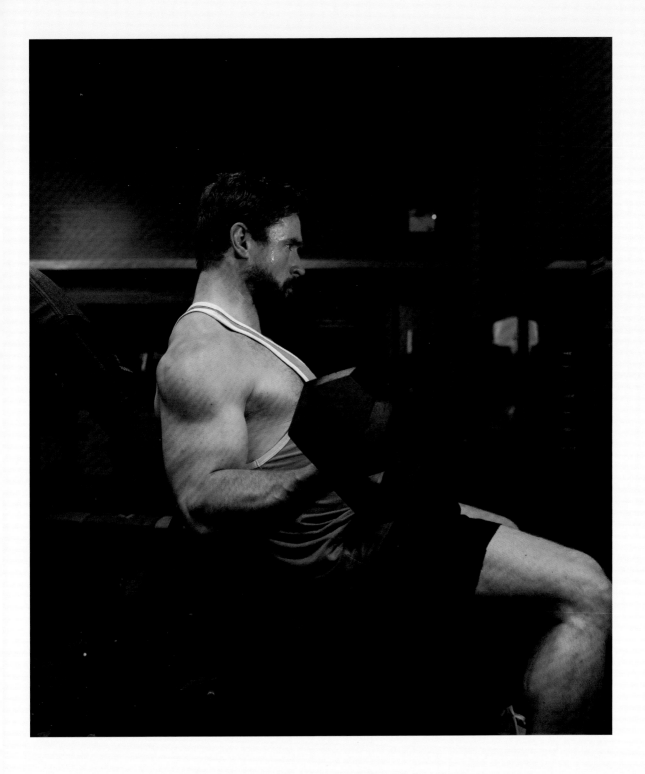

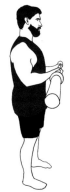

Barbell bicep curls

- Stand upright with a barbell in your hands, palms facing forwards and hands shoulder-width apart.
- Keep your elbows close to your sides and your core engaged.
- Curl the barbell upwards towards your shoulders by bending your elbows, keeping your upper arms stationary.
- Squeeze your biceps at the top of the movement.
- Slowly lower the barbell back down to the starting position.

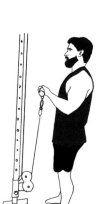

Cable bicep curls

- Attach a straight or angled bar to a low pulley on a cable machine.
- Stand facing the machine and grip the bar with both hands, palms facing upwards.
- Keep your elbows close to your sides and your core engaged.
- Curl the bar upwards towards your shoulders by bending your elbows, keeping your upper arms stationary.
- Squeeze your biceps at the top of the movement.
- Slowly lower the bar back down to the starting position.

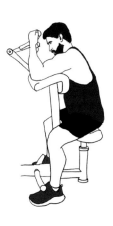

Machine bicep curls

- Adjust the seat and handles of the machine to fit your body comfortably.
- Sit down on the machine and grip the handles with your palms facing upwards.
- Keep your elbows close to your sides and your core engaged.
- Curl the handles upwards towards your shoulders by bending your elbows, keeping your upper arms stationary.
- Squeeze your biceps at the top of the movement.
- Slowly lower the handles back down to the starting position.

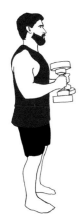

Dumbbell hammer curls

- Stand upright with a dumbbell in each hand, arms fully extended by your sides, palms facing in towards your body (neutral grip).
- Keep your elbows close to your sides and your core engaged.
- Curl the dumbbells upwards towards your shoulders by bending your elbows, keeping your palms facing inwards throughout the movement.
- Squeeze your biceps at the top of the movement.
- Slowly lower the dumbbells back down to the starting position.

Cable hammer curls

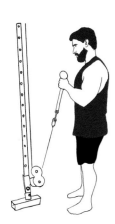

- Attach a rope handle to a low pulley on a cable machine.
- Stand facing the machine and grip the rope with both hands, palms facing in towards your body (neutral grip).
- Keep your elbows close to your sides and your core engaged.
- Curl the rope upwards towards your shoulders by bending your elbows, keeping your palms facing inwards throughout the movement.
- Squeeze your biceps at the top of the movement.
- Slowly lower the rope back down to the starting position.

Machine hammer curls

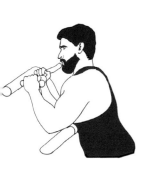

- Adjust the seat and handles of the machine to fit your body comfortably.
- Sit down on the machine and grip the handles with both hands, palms facing in towards your body (neutral grip).
- Keep your elbows close to your sides and your core engaged.
- Curl the handles upwards towards your shoulders by bending your elbows, keeping your palms facing inwards throughout the movement.
- Squeeze your biceps at the top of the movement.
- Slowly lower the handles back down to the starting position.

Accessory (lower body)

Machine seated leg curl

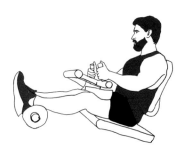

- Adjust the machine seat and leg pad to fit your body comfortably.
- Sit down on the machine with your back against the backrest and your legs extended in front of you.
- Place your lower legs under the leg pad, just above your ankles.
- Grip the handles of the machine for stability.
- Flex your knees to curl the leg pad towards your glutes, contracting your hamstrings.
- Keep your upper body stable throughout the movement.
- Pause briefly at the top of the movement, then slowly lower the leg pad back to the starting position.

Machine lying leg curl

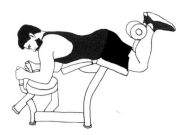

- Adjust the machine to fit your body comfortably.
- Lie face down on the machine with your knees just off the edge of the bench and your legs fully extended.
- Position your ankles under the leg pad, just above your heels.
- Grip the handles of the machine for stability.
- Flex your knees to curl the leg pad towards your glutes, contracting your hamstrings.
- Keep your hips pressed into the bench and your upper body relaxed throughout the movement.
- Pause briefly at the top of the movement, then slowly lower the leg pad back to the starting position.

Machine leg extension

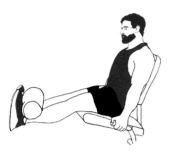

- Adjust the machine seat and leg pad to fit your body comfortably.
- Sit down on the machine with your back against the backrest and your legs extended in front of you.
- Place your lower legs under the leg pad, just above your ankles.
- Grip the handles of the machine for stability.
- Extend your knees to lift the leg pad upwards, straightening your legs.
- Keep your upper body stable throughout the movement.
- Pause briefly at the top of the movement, then slowly lower the leg pad back to the starting position.

Machine standing calf raises

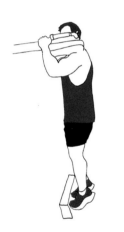

- Adjust the machine to fit your body comfortably.
- Stand on the machine with the balls of your feet on the foot platform and your heels hanging off the edge.
- Hold on to the handles of the machine for stability.
- Rise up onto your tiptoes by lifting your heels as high as possible.
- Squeeze your calf muscles at the top of the movement.
- Lower your heels back down towards the starting position, allowing them to drop below the level of the foot platform to stretch your calves.

Machine bent-knee calf raises

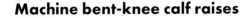

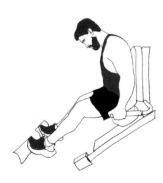

- Adjust the machine to fit your body comfortably.
- Sit down on the machine with your back against the backrest and your knees bent at a 90-degree angle.
- Place the balls of your feet on the foot platform so that your heels are hanging off the edge.
- Hold on to the handles of the machine for stability.
- Rise up onto your tiptoes by lifting your heels as high as possible.
- Squeeze your calf muscles at the top of the movement.
- Lower your heels back down towards the starting position, allowing them to drop below the level of the foot platform to stretch your calves.

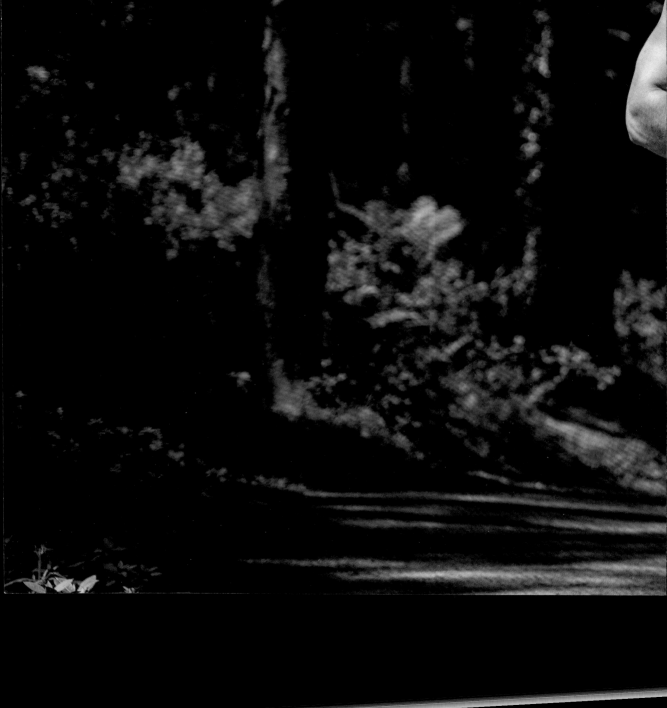

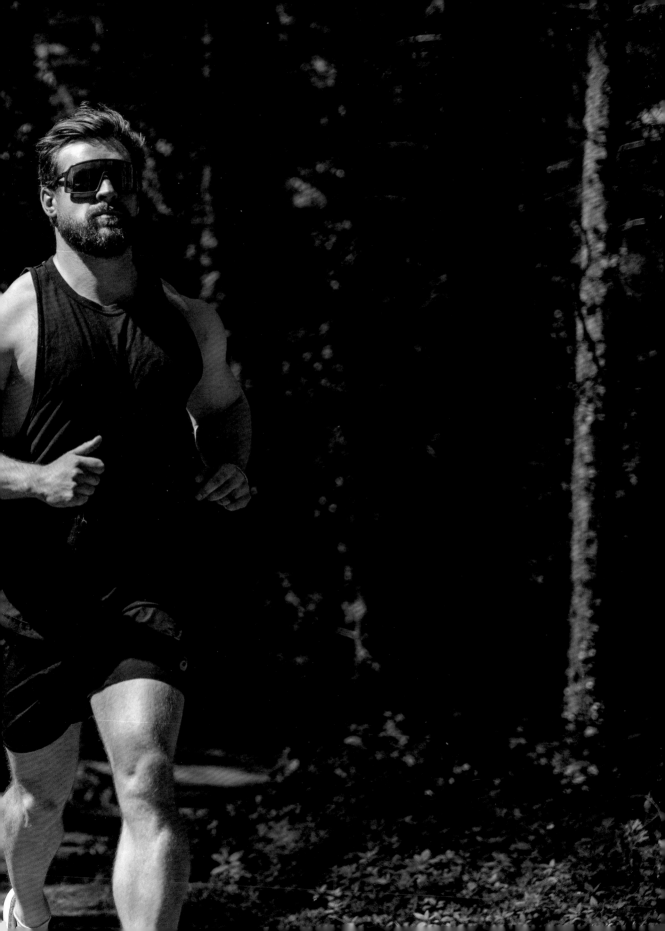

AFTERWORD

In 2018 I received a golden ticket from Dwayne 'The Rock' Johnson to compete for a spot in *The Titan Games*. *The Titan Games* was an American TV show (airing in 2019 and 2020) in which very fit people competed against each other through a series of gruelling challenges to test their physical fitness, strength and grit. The sixty-four contestants who took part in the show were selected from a larger pool of three hundred people.

I was one of those three hundred people. When I received the invitation, I was incredibly excited. But as I walked onto the set, I felt a surge of imposter syndrome. Everyone around me looked so big and strong. (And tall. Some of these pro athletes were over six and a half feet tall, towering over my 5'8" frame.) I couldn't help thinking, 'What the heck am I doing here?' But I did my best to quell that voice and concentrate on the task at hand.

The organisers sorted us into groups of ten. From there, we competed against each other in a series of tests including a broad (long) jump, a vertical (high) jump, an obstacle course, a deadlift, an infinite monkey bar climb (on an incline) and a treadmill run (again, on an increasing incline).

I did well throughout the day, and my imposter syndrome eased off as I found that I could hold my own against these mega-athletes, many of whom played professional sports or had served in the upper echelons of the US military. I nearly had the best broad jump of the bunch, coming second only to someone who was half a foot taller than me. My hands looked like raw tuna by the time I finished the monkey bar challenge, but I managed to get the joint top score within my group. The inner voice that told me I didn't belong had no choice but to quiet in the face of my results. The proof was in the pudding: I was just as good than my competitors, and they were among the best of the best.

And then the running challenge commenced. We entered a room stacked with treadmills. As we ran, the speed and the incline increased. This was a 'last one standing' challenge, meaning the goal was to simply keep running longer than everyone else. I was situated in the front row, which meant I couldn't see my competitors other than those directly to my left or right. But I could hear them. And the longer I ran, the quieter things got as the treadmills around me stopped. Bit by bit, my competitors quit. After what seemed like hours (but was probably thirty minutes in total), the person on my right, a big, jacked, ex-special ops military dude, finally called it quits. Then the person on my left, an ex-pro football player for Penn State, gave up. At a certain point, my legs went numb. A metallic taste coated my throat and tongue, and I was covered in sweat. The incline was so steep I could barely get my legs high enough to meet it. But still, I kept running. Finally, one of the organisers came over and told me, 'That's it, Ben. It's over. You won.'

I collapsed on the ground. I couldn't think. I could barely breathe. But I was flooded with happiness and an overwhelming sense of relief that my CF hadn't dictated my results. I felt that I was increasing the gap between myself and that CF Terminator. *I did it.* Somehow I had got myself here, to this point, where I could outrun and outlast some of the fittest people around.

If you happened to watch *The Titan Games*, you'll know I didn't get to be on the show. Unfortunately, the producers weren't able to secure a visa for me to work in the US, so I wasn't able to participate. This was incredibly disappointing, since I clearly had the physical capability to compete. The producers and my fellow competitors were incredibly supportive of me and my story; they couldn't believe I had cystic fibrosis. (And remember, this was before the new triple combination therapy medications emerged in the UK market.) I had wanted so badly to share my story with the world and show people what someone with CF was capable of. Needless to say, I was crushed.

But as I returned home, my disappointment faded and something new emerged in its place. A sense of peace came over me. That Terminator-like voice that represented my worst fears about myself and my health had gone silent. I felt like I'd Spartan-kicked it so far away it couldn't touch me. For once, I felt truly limitless.

As I reflected on my physical performance and all the challenges I'd competed, I thought, *imagine that.* If only I could have known, as I sat in that

Keep showing up. Using this book as your guide, take small actions every chance you get. If you slip up or make mistakes, shrug them off as best you can and keep on going.

hospital room all those years ago while the cystic fibrosis specialist told me my lung function might never improve, that not only would my lung function get better, but one day I would be outperforming elite athletes and military professionals. I almost wish I could go back and tell myself just how good things would get. I'm not sure my younger self would have believed it.

Certainly, if my sixteen-year-old self could have seen photos or videos of me today, he would have been convinced he was being pranked. Frankly, it's still hard for me to believe that, over the course of fifteen years, I've gained 27 kilos (60 lbs) of muscle (nearly half my body weight from where I started). And I gained it all one pound at a time.

Honestly, if I had a time machine, I would go back and thank my sixteen-year-old self. I am so thankful for him. I'm thankful he kept going out to the garage to use the workout machine on those cold winter mornings, when it was so damp and chilly he could see his breath in the air, and the plates were almost too cold to touch. His friends wouldn't come and join him because it was too cold, but he did it anyway.

I'm also thankful for my twenty-two-year-old self who asked for a stationary bike while stuck in the hospital. And for the version of me who left the hospital absolutely determined to get his lung function back. I'm thankful to him for all the times he kept showing up, even when he was hesitant, disappointed, fearful or downright terrified. I'm thankful for the way my past self was brave enough to challenge all the limitations I grew up with – both real and perceived. I'm thankful for his determination to keep outrunning his inner Terminator, and his utter refusal to be held back by cystic fibrosis. I'm endlessly thankful for his commitment to living a limitless life.

Of course, I owe a debt of gratitude to the many people who have supported me in this journey. I am deeply appreciative of each of them. But there's no better feeling than being able to look back and thank yourself for doing the work that brought you to where you are today.

If you're reading this, I want you to know that this same feeling – the feeling that you've become the person you want to be, and have your previous self to thank – is possible. That person you want to be? They're out there, waiting for you. To bring them into existence, all you have to do is start. Do what they would do. Act the way they would act. Be the person you want to be, one small effort at a time.

In this book, I've covered the basic principles of good health and fitness: sleep, mental health, nutrition, movement and resistance training. As I've said throughout, none of this is particularly sexy. It's all bread-and-butter stuff. But these efforts provide the foundation for everything and anything. The better you get at them, the more confidence you'll have. And that confidence will flow into other areas of your life. Your work, your relationships, your sense of who you are – everything will benefit. Confidence is like gold dust, and as it grows within you, everything in your life will shimmer.

So that's my final piece of advice: keep showing up. Using this book as your guide, take small actions every chance you get. If you slip up or make mistakes, shrug them off as best you can and keep on going. Trust me on this: imperfect actions will always beat perfect intentions. Don't worry if your efforts aren't perfect, or if you think you aren't there yet. Keep moving in the direction you want to go, towards that person you want to be.

In time, you'll look back and thank yourself. You'll know that, thanks to all your small efforts, the possibilities are endless. You'll know, without a doubt, that you are truly limitless.

ACKNOWLEDGMENTS

This book wouldn't exist without the following people, who I will be forever grateful to.

A special thank you to my wife and best friend, Janice. Your unwavering support, patience and love have been the cornerstone of this journey. Your

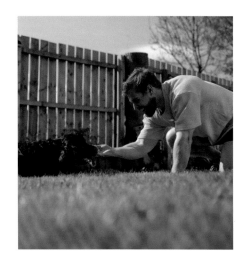

encouragement and your belief in me when I doubt myself make all the difference. Thank you for always being my rock, my sounding board and my greatest cheerleader from the beginning.

To my family and friends who have supported me throughout every idea and adventure, always cheering me along. A special thanks to my talented friend Chris McCann, who captured the images for this book. It wouldn't look the same without them.

To the Little, Brown team who made this book possible and have been so encouraging and supportive from start to finish: Ed, Alex and Nithya, and to Sian and Emil at D.R. ink for making it look so good.

To Camille DePutter for the many conference calls and taking all my thoughts, stories and ideas and putting them into text. Camille's skills were invaluable and allowed me to share my journey with you, which is something I honestly thought would just remain as a collection of random notes on my phone.

I want to say a massive thanks to all my clients: thank you for trusting me with your health and fitness journey and allowing me to do the best job in the world.

Finally to you (*the one reading this*), thank you for supporting me through this book. I hope it helps you to live life without limits.